The Essential Guide to Coding in Audiology

Coding, Billing, and Practice Management

Editor-in-Chief for Audiology
Brad A. Stach, PhD

The Essential Guide to Coding in Audiology

Coding, Billing, and Practice Management

Debra Abel, AuD

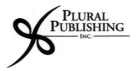

PLURAL
PUBLISHING
INC.

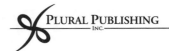

5521 Ruffin Road
San Diego, CA 92123
e-mail: info@pluralpublishing.com
Website: http://www.pluralpublishing.com

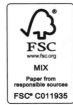

Typeset in 11/13 Palatino Roman by Achorn International.
Printed in the United States of America by McNaughton & Gunn.

Library of Congress Cataloging-in-Publication Data

Names: Abel, Debra, editor.
Title: The essential guide to coding in audiology : coding, billing, and
 practice management / [edited by] Debra Abel.
Description: San Diego, CA : Plural Publishing [2018] | Includes
 bibliographical references and index.
Identifiers: LCCN 2017030923 | ISBN 9781597568937 (alk. paper) |
 ISBN 1597568937 (alk. paper)
Subjects: | MESH: Audiology—organization & administration | Clinical
 Coding | Reimbursement Mechanisms | Practice Management,
 Medical | Government Regulation
Classification: LCC RF291.3 | NLM WV 21 | DDC 617.80076—dc23
LC record available at https://lccn.loc.gov/2017030923

Contents

Foreword

There has never been a more crucial time in the profession of audiology for a book on coding and reimbursement. Numerous changes have impacted reimbursement for audiology in the last several years: increased health care regulation, cutbacks for audiologists' services both diagnostic and rehabilitative, inconsistencies in payment between insurance providers, and the list goes on and on. Coding knowledge must be part of every audiologist's diet. Knowledge of coding helps increase your revenue. No knowledge of coding and you just might starve. It often seems like running in a maze. So "yes," this is a perfect time for a book on coding and reimbursement.

I am grateful to Dr. Abel who has been so passionate about the topic of reimbursement. Thanks to her leadership she has been able to move this reimbursement agenda forward. Dr. Abel has had a wealth of experience in coding and reimbursement throughout her career so this makes her the perfect choice as author and editor. Her career journey in this area includes:

- Owning a private practice in Alliance, Ohio where she first became frustrated with lack of audiology reimbursement
- 1980–1990 Member of the Ohio Governmental Affairs Committee (GAC) working on audiology reimbursement
- 1999–2000 Chair of the Coding and Reimbursement Committee for the American Academy of Audiology
- 2007–2015 Appointed to the position of Director of Reimbursement for the American Academy of Audiology
- 2008 Chapter "Coding, Billing, and Reimbursement Capture" in Glaser and Traynor, *Strategic Practice Management: A Patient-Centric Approach*
- 2014 Chapter "Coding, Reimbursement, and Practice Management" in Glaser and Traynor, *Strategic Practice Management: Business and Procedural Considerations,* Second Edition

Dr. Abel has provided a brilliant list of interesting highly qualified contributors each providing an exhaustive litany of valuable, relevant, and current information never before assembled in a single work. Dr. Abel begins the comprehensive text with two chapters beginning with a thorough discussion of various codes: CPT®, ICD-10, CM, and HCPCS, and a detailed guidance on Medicare billing.

Dr. Doug Lewis writing on "Federal Regulations Applicable to Audiology" will likely be viewed as the best treatise on the topic written in our field to date. He has hit the mark with well-developed clarity. Dr. Kim Cavitt writes on "Third-Party Reimbursement, Contracting, and Credentialing for Audiology Services." Dr. Cavitt provides an excellent review and delineation necessary for contract negotiations and optimal credentialing. She clarifies that it is the growth of hearing aids that has made the stakes higher and the need to understand third-party payers, contracting, and credentialing. Dr. Stephanie Sjoblad writes on "Itemizing Professional Services for Hearing Aids." She provides a brilliant discussion comparing "unbundling" and "itemizing" and includes an outstanding list of references. Kim Pollock, R.N., writes on "Practicing in an Otolaryngology Office: Understanding Your Role in the Revenue Cycle." She provides noteworthy tables and figures as well as reviewing Explanations and Benefits (EOB) documents.

This team of contributors' knowledge and expertise are, quite frankly, unsurpassed. Without question this book will provide a format others in various healthcare disciplines will likely emulate. There is clarity in every keystroke! For the practice of audiology to thrive in the current tumult that is health care, understanding coding and reimbursement is essential. This book lays the foundation for that success.

Robert G. Glaser, PhD
Past President, American Academy of Audiology

Introduction

This book was written only by audiologists for audiologists as a guide to bill and be reimbursed for the hearing and balance services performed within the framework of the required federal and state regulations applicable to audiologists. The goal of this book is to provide contemporary information and the supporting resources in one location for what may seem to be elusive information for audiologists as well as for students regarding coding, reimbursement, and compliance processes facing audiologists in most settings. At press time, there were no other coding and compliance books written exclusively for audiologists.

Coding and compliance is a dynamic process and to assist, a toolbox of the three code families vital to audiologists is detailed within these pages. The procedure codes (CPT® codes) utilized by audiologists are offered with their Relative Value Units and should be used in conjunction with guidance from the American Medical Association (AMA) and the Centers for Medicare and Medicaid Services (CMS) as was done in the writing of this book. Both the disease codes (ICD-10 codes), current at press time, and the HCPCS codes for hearing aids and related services utilized by audiologists, found in the public sector, for example, the Internet, are also provided here so that the reader can have these at their fingertips in order to save time and effort. For options regarding hearing aid billing, insights into the world of insurance and contracts, understanding your revenue cycle, and the specifics of the laws that pertain to practicing audiologists and students, the readers only need to look so far as the other chapters.

Contributors

Debra Abel, AuD
Contracting Services
Audigy
Poway, California

Kimberly M. Cavitt, AuD
Audiology Resources, Inc.
Northwestern University
Chicago, Illinois

Douglas A. Lewis, JD, PhD, AuD, MBA
Excalibur Business Consultants/Excalibur
  Entertainment
Private Practice Healthcare Solutions
Dublin, Ohio

Kimberley J. Pollock, RN, MBA, CPC, CMDP
KarenZupko & Associates, Inc.
Chicago, Illinois

Stephanie Sjoblad, AuD
UNC Hearing & Communication Center
University of North Carolina at Chapel Hill
  School of Medicine
Chapel Hill, North Carolina

Acknowledgments

In writing this book, I'd like to acknowledge the talents and expertise of those who have contributed chapters: Kim Cavitt, Doug Lewis, Kim Pollack, and Stephanie Sjoblad. I've had the personal experience and joy of collaborating with them either in print or in presentations and am very honored they agreed to be a part of this project.

There are always people to thank at times like this and I'd like to take the opportunity to thank the following for their expertise, guidance, support, and in nearly all cases, their lengthy friendship.

Robert Glaser, PhD, the co-author of *Strategic Practice Management,* has been the mentor we all should be fortunate to have. As chair of the Coding and Reimbursement Committee of the American Academy of Audiology in the 1980s, Bob placed me on the committee, the next year appointed me as his co-chair, which then led to being the chair, then as the Board staff liaison, and then staff. By including me in his book, it eventually led to this one based on the direction of his insight. In addition, I'd like to thank Kim Pollock who lured me to write the audiology chapter in *The Essential Guide to Coding in Otolaryngology,* which also led to this. Audiology friends who have always been supportive along the way, Kim Cavitt, Tom Hutchison, Jane Kukula, Marilyn Larkin, Lisa Satterfield, Jennifer Shinn, and Therese Walden have been there during compelling times, always encouraging and supportive.

I'd like to also recognize Mike Halloran, my boss at Audigy, who has been an immense support in this new phase of my career. Finally, there wouldn't be a book if it wasn't for the American Academy of Audiology, the personal incubator for learning all things coding, reimbursement, and compliance related, who allowed me to serve them and learn for nearly 8 years.

On a very personal note I must acknowledge my late husband, Ted Abel, my greatest life rudder, supporter, and encourager. For so many years, he showed many of us how to live a life which exuded courage and provided inspiration in the most difficult of times.

The profession is experiencing dynamic and unprecedented times. In June 2016, the National Academies of Sciences, Engineering and Medicine's (NASEM) Committee on Accessible and Affordable Hearing Health Care for Adults released their report of 12 recommended actions that have and will impact the way audiologists provide services to patients. These chapters hope to offer the essential tools in navigating these uncharted waters.

CHAPTER 1

The Codes: CPT®, ICD-10-CM, and HCPCS Necessary to Bill Audiology Services

Debra Abel

Introduction

This initial chapter describes the foundation and tools for reimbursement, the codes for the services provided within the scope of practice of an audiologist. This alphabet soup includes the Current Procedural Terminology (CPT®) codes, the procedures; the International Classification of Diseases (ICD-10-CM) or diseases and diagnoses codes used in private practice and physician practice offices (ICD-10-PCS applies to inpatient hospital services and is not included in this chapter); and the Healthcare Common Procedural Coding System (HCPCS II) codes which include hearing aid related services and several procedure codes, FM/DM system codes, assistive listening device codes, and cochlear implant and osseo integrated codes for devices and replacement parts. Each claim must have CPT® and/or HCPCS codes and at least one ICD-10 code in order to be filed. A diagnostic/disease code should be chosen based on the reason for the test, the signs and symptoms the patient relays to you, and should be included in the patient's record, and/or the outcome of the test results.

To understand the process and necessity of correctly coding and billing for audiologic services, it's important to remember they are not only the vehicle for payment, but are also used for tracking purposes. Medicare serves as the benchmark for many health care providers due to the imposed requirements, the most defined regulations applicable to audiologists; commercial payers may follow the same guidelines. Medicare tracks this coding information and policies are created in response, especially when professional trends may occur (e.g., a significant increase in utilization of a procedure over several years). This is what led to the 2012 revised description of CPT Code 92540, which required the bundling of procedures performed on the same date of service, thereby reducing the reimbursement due to the elimination of pre-, intra-, and post-service times that are included within the code's valuation. Additionally, Medicare tracks what is known as outliers, those providers who bill differently than their collegial counterparts for the same services, which may trigger an audit. The next chapter will discuss Medicare requirements in greater detail, but briefly, to understand the foundation of the regulations which impact performing and billing Medicare diagnostic audiology procedures, the Centers for Medicare and Medicaid Services (CMS) Program Memorandum AB-02-080 states "diagnostic testing, including hearing and balance assessment services, performed by a qualified audiologist is paid for as 'other diagnostic tests' under §1861 (s)

1

(3) of the Social Security Act (the Act) when a physician orders testing to obtain information as part of his/her diagnostic evaluation or to determine the appropriate medical or surgical treatment of a hearing deficit or related medical problem" (CMS, 2002). This section is the reason why Medicare recognizes audiologists only for diagnostic testing procedures and why a physician order is required. It would literally take an act of Congress to change these requirements.

Diagnostic audiologic services provided under the "other diagnostic test" category in section 1861(s)(3) of the Social Security Act are not to be billed as "incident to" services to Medicare. In 2008, the CMS issued Transmittal 84, which required all audiologists to bill services supplied to Medicare Part B beneficiaries under their own National Provider Identifier (NPI) and not by way of the NPI of a physician. Unfortunately, this practice of billing audiology services performed by an audiologist and billed by an otolaryngologist continues and if discovered, Medicare will likely seek repayments as well as penalties and interest.

At the time of publication, Medicare recognizes audiologists only as diagnosticians, not providers of treatment of hearing and balance disorders such as the rehabilitation of hearing loss, tinnitus management, and management of those experiencing imbalance disorders. Although more restrictive in scope than state licensure laws, which define a provider's scope of practice allowing diagnosis and treatment, some payers do recognize and reimburse for all professional services that audiologists are licensed to provide. It behooves a practice to be aware of the differences in requirements for audiological services among payers.

Key Procedure Codes

As with any provider of health care services, audiologists utilize Current Procedural Terminology (CPT®), International Classification of Disease (ICD), and Healthcare Common Procedure Coding System II (HCPCS) codes. Specific HCPCS II codes include the L section for osseointegrated devices and the V section related to hearing aid technology, dispensing fees, assistive listening devices, and a few hearing aid related procedures. Under

the Medicine/Special Otorhinolaryngological Services section of CPT®, the codes utilized by audiologists include the following categories and will be detailed in the next section:

- Vestibular function
- Audiologic function
- Evaluation/assessment services

All CPT® codes utilized by audiologists are for both ears unless a modifier is utilized (e.g., 52, or RT, LT as indicated by the payer).

Each coding system will be discussed in order to serve as a common basis of understanding what is required when filing a claim that must include CPT® and/or HCPCS code(s) and ICD-10 codes.

Definition of CPT® Codes

Vestibular Function Tests (92537-92546, 92548)

Introduction – CPT® codes 92537-92546 and 92548 have separate technical and professional components. Medicare requires the testing to be billed under the NPI of the performing audiologist and the code is reported without any modifiers; this is called global billing. A technician may perform the technical component of the test and the physician providing direct supervision will bill the code with modifier TC to Medicare, known as "incident to" billing. Either the audiologist or the physician may perform the interpretation and report and would bill the code with modifier 26 for the professional component. Audiologists cannot bill "incident to" for another provider, only themselves. For all tests, a printout and the interpretation of the test results should be included in the patient's medical record.

Vestibular Codes

1. Basic vestibular evaluation (92540)
   a. *Definition* – CPT® 92540 includes 92541, 92542, 92544, and 92545. For electronystagmography (ENG), vertical electrodes (+92547) are applied and are billed as one unit per date of service.

Eye movements are tracked with a light stimulus, and eye movement is evaluated upward, downward, and side to side, looking for the presence of nystagmus.
   b. *Key points* – Do not report 92540 with any of the four tests listed above. If only 1 to 3 of these are performed on the same date of service, use modifier 59 (distinct procedural service) on the lower valued separate codes and include in the documentation why the tests were performed (National Correct Coding Initiative [NCCI] 2015).
2. Caloric vestibular test with recording, bilateral; bithermal (i.e., one warm and one cool irrigation in each ear for a total of four irrigations) (92537).
3. 92538 monothermal (i.e., one irrigation in each ear for a total of two irrigations)
   a. *Definition* – The caloric vestibular test is performed by irrigating the ear canal with either warm or cool water or air, then recording the eye movement response (nystagmus).
   b. *Key points* – 92537 will be billed with one unit when performing the four irrigations and 92538 will be billed with one unit when performing the two irrigations.
4. Sinusoidal vertical axis rotational testing (92546)
   a. For CPT® 92546 the use of a computer controlled rotary chair is used to evaluate nystagmus with the patient, wearing electrodes, seated with their head bent forward with their eyes closed.
   b. Some payers are requesting the serial number of the chair in order to ensure that correct billing for the procedure by the appropriate provider has occurred.
5. Computerized Dynamic Posturography (92548)
   a. *Definition* – For CPT® 92548, the patient stands, secured in a harness on a computer-controlled platform equipped with sensors that examine the patient's reaction and adjustments to body movements generated by the platform's movements.
   b. *Key points* – Several tests, including the Sensory Organization Test (SOT), are included.

Audiologic Function Tests

The following audiological tests do not have separate professional and technical components; there-fore, they may not be performed by a technician and billed to Medicare under a supervising physician's or audiologist's NPI. As with all testing, a printout and the interpretation of the test results should be included in the patient's medical record.

1. Tympanometry and reflex threshold measurements (92550)
   a. *Definition* – CPT® 92550 includes tympanometry and acoustic reflexes, ipsilaterally and contralaterally for multiple frequencies bilaterally.
   b. *Key points* – if performing only ipsilateral or only contralateral reflexes, use modifier 52 to indicate that the entire procedure was not completed.
2. Comprehensive audiometry threshold evaluation and speech recognition (92557)
   a. *Definition* – This includes otoscopy, pure tone air and bone conduction, speech reception thresholds, and word recognition scores.
   b. *Key points* – This code includes 92553 and 92556 which should not be billed separately. Often when hearing acuity is within normal limits, bone conduction is not performed and if so, 92557 should be appended with the -52 modifier to indicate reduced services.
3. Evoked optoacoustic emissions, screening (qualitative measurement of distortion product or transient evoked otoacoustic emissions), automated analysis (92558)
   a. *Definition* – This is often utilized for newborn infant hearing screening, typically with automated equipment at 1 dB level, resulting in a pass or refer.
   b. *Key points* – This code has 0 wRVUs and is a non-covered service by Medicare and often by commercial payers.
4. Tympanometry (impedance testing) (92567)
   a. *Definition* – This test of middle ear pressure is performed by inserting a probe tip into the ear canal, securing a seal, and then introducing positive and negative pressure to move the tympanic membrane. This determines normal versus pathologic conditions often described by Jerger Types A, B, C, As, and Ad.
   b. *Key points* – There is no definitive coding guidance if a seal cannot be obtained or maintained, but proof of attempts in the documentation should be noted; modifier 52 is suggested when this occurs.

5. Acoustic immittance testing includes tympanometry (impedance testing), acoustic reflex threshold testing, and acoustic reflex decay testing (92570)
   a. *Definition* – This includes tympanometry and acoustic reflex thresholds, ipsilaterally and contralaterally and acoustic reflex decay at 500 and 1000 Hz, bilaterally, 10 dB higher than the acoustic reflex threshold at those specific frequencies.
   b. *Key points* – If performing only ipsilateral or only contralateral reflexes, append modifier 52 to indicate that the entire procedure was not completed. The presence of acoustic reflex decay indicates further testing or consultations with other health care professionals.

6. Visual reinforcement audiometry (VRA) (92579)
   a. *Definition* – This test includes obtaining both tonal or speech information using speakers or earphones, with the head-turning response reinforced by the use of moving toys, flashing lights, and/or video.
   b. *Key Points* – This is typically utilized with the pediatric, cognitively impaired, and/or nonverbal populations

7. Conditioning play audiometry (92582)
   a. *Definition* – This too is typically utilized with the pediatric population; they are taught and conditioned to drop a block or a toy in a box when they hear a sound or a similar activity, usually presented via earphones.
   b. *Key points* – Speech detection or reception thresholds can be filed separately (e.g., 92555) as speech testing is not included in this code.

8. Auditory Evoked Potentials for evoked response audiometry and/or testing of the central nervous system; comprehensive (92585)
   a. *Definition* – This neurophysiological test is used as a site of lesion test for acoustic neuromas and other neurological diagnoses, view neural effects which may include toxins that can impact the central auditory pathway, assist in the diagnosis of auditory neuropathy, and serve as a test of threshold detection. A series of waveforms is produced and classified based on wave morphology, time, intensity, and latencies.
   b. *Key points* – Electrodes are required and are part of the test protocol, with no separate reporting of any code, for example, 92547. A printout of the test result should be included in the patient's record.

9. Distortion product evoked otoacoustic emissions, limited evaluation (to confirm the presence or absence of hearing disorder, 3 to 6 frequencies), or transient evoked otoacoustic emissions, with interpretation and report (92587)
   a. *Definition* – This test to verify cochlear outer hair cell function is typically used to evaluate differentiate cochlear versus retrocochlear function in those with asymmetric hearing loss, for monitoring cochlear status in those patients exposed to an ototoxic agent, and those difficult to test such as infants, toddlers, developmentally delayed, and/or malingerers.
   b. *Key points* – If using Distortion Product Otoacoustic Emissions (DPOAEs), 3 to 6 frequencies must be tested in each ear, with interpretation and report. Transient Evoked Otoacoustic Emissions are also accepted for use when filing this code.

10. Comprehensive diagnostic evaluation (quantitative analysis of outer hair cell function by cochlear mapping, minimum of 12 frequencies), with interpretation and report (92588)
    a. Definition – A minimum of 12 frequencies in each ear are tested for a total of 24 bilaterally.
    b. Key points – This is typically performed for tinnitus and/or ototoxicity monitoring, pediatric testing, and cochlear versus retrocochlear lesion differential diagnosis to determine cochlear outer hair cell function.

Audiology Function Tests with Separate Technical and Professional Components

Unlike the audiologic function tests in the previous section, codes 92585, 92587, and 92588 have separate technical and professional components utilized similarly to the technical and professional components associated with the vestibular tests. Medicare permits a technician to perform the test and the physician who provides the required direct supervision to bill the code with the TC modifier. Either the audiologist or the physician may perform the interpretation and report for the same test and would then bill the code with the 26 modifier for the professional component. If the audiologist performed the test, the interpretation, and the report, then the claim is filed with the global code (no modifiers) under the NPI of the audiologist. As with the other tests discussed, a printout and the interpretation of the test results should be included in the patient's medical record.

Evaluative and Therapeutic Services

The following codes are for common evaluation and assessment services performed by audiologists.

1. Evaluation of central auditory function, with report; initial 60 minutes (92620)
   a. *Definition* – This battery of tests includes auditory figure-ground tests, tonal pattern recognition, competing words, speech in noise, and tonal duration.
   b. *Key points* – The beginning and end times of the face-to-face evaluation should be included in the chart documentation, as this is a test for the initial 60 minutes. If additional time is required, each 15 minute block can be billed with CPT® 92621. The reduced services modifier, 52, does not apply to time-based codes. If the procedure was 30 minutes or less, CPT® code 92700 (unlisted otorhinolaryngological service or procedure) may be utilized, likely requiring supporting documentation.
2. Assessment of tinnitus (includes pitch, loudness matching, and masking) (92625)
   a. *Definition* – This code requires three distinct procedures when evaluating patients with tinnitus (self-perceived sounds). This includes: pitch, loudness matching, and masking. The patient is to match the type of tinnitus when stimuli are offered in a bracketing method as well as for the intensity of their tinnitus. Once established, minimum masking levels are introduced for one minute to determine if the patient experienced a change in their tinnitus.
3. Evaluation of auditory rehabilitation status; first hour (92626)
   a. *Definition* – this assesses the effectiveness of a patient's residual hearing either prior to or after receiving monaural or binaural hearing aids, cochlear implants, osseointegrated devices, and/or a brainstem implant. The audiologist determines auditory rehabilitation status with

a series of speech-perception (speech awareness, speech recognition, sound discrimination, and speech in noise) and communication outcome measures, prior to any therapeutic intervention, to determine the need for any therapies and to monitor progress.
   b. *Key Points* – This is not a counseling code nor does it include hearing aid examination and selection, hearing aid fitting, or the cochlear implant programming codes (see 92601-92604). The times when the face-to-face evaluation began and ended should be included in the chart documentation. CPT® code 92626 should not be used if the procedure lasted less than 31 minutes. If the procedure was 30 minutes or less, CPT® code 92700 (unlisted otorhinolaryngological service or procedure) may be utilized, likely requiring supporting documentation. The reduced services modifier, 52, does not apply to time-based codes, and thus cannot be used. If this requires more than one hour of time, then 92627 can be billed for each additional 15-minute time period.
4. Diagnostic analysis of cochlear implant, patient younger than 7 years of age, with programming and subsequent reprogramming and diagnostic analysis of cochlear implant, age 7 years or older, with programming and subsequent reprogramming (92601-92604).

   Also included in the Evaluative and Therapeutic Services section are the four CPT® cochlear implant codes (92601-92604), the choice of which is based on age as well as the device status of either being stimulated initially or for subsequent mapping. For those cochlear implant patients younger than 7 years of age, the initial implant stimulation is 92601 and for subsequent programming/mapping for the same aged patient, 92602. For those age 7 or older, the initial stimulation of the implants is 92603 and for subsequent reprogramming/mapping, 92604.
5. Unlisted otorhinolaryngological service or procedure (92700)
   a. *Definition* – When there is not a dedicated CPT® code describing a service provided, as in the question posed in the March 2011 CPT® Assistant regarding coding for Vestibular Evoked Myogenic Potentials (VEMPs), an unlisted code may be reported.

b. *Key points* – A narrative describing the procedure and accompanying literature demonstrating its validity should be submitted when a denial is issued.

Key Modifiers

There are times during the course of providing services that the procedure doesn't transpire as it is typically required, such as with pediatric and demented patients or with patients when only one ear is tested or if not all the tests of a bundled code are completed. The following modifiers indicate to the payer that these services are altered. Many payers do not recognize some of these modifiers, but it is still necessary to append them when there is a change to the provision of the service.

22   Increased Procedural Services
This can be used during an evaluation that requires additional testing such as when a child or an adult with dementia is distracted during the testing and needs to be reminded of how and when to respond, resulting in an increase of time and complexity of the procedure. The use of this code may result in a denial, in which case the chart notes detailing what was done and why it took longer than the typical procedure will be helpful in the appeal.

26   Professional Component
This is used when only the interpretation and report are performed for a code that has both the professional and technical components (e.g., 92537-92546, 92548, 92585, 92587, and 92588). For example, the audiologist provides only the professional component, only doing the interpretation and creating the report of a basic vestibular evaluation (92540-26).

TC   Technical Component
This is used when only the technical aspect is performed for any of the codes categorized with technical and professional components (e.g., 92537-92546, 92548, 92585, 92587, and 92588). For example, if the audiologist provides only the technical component of a basic vestibular evaluation by performing only the testing, the service would be filed with 92540-TC by the audiologist. For those audiologists employed in an otolaryngology practice, if the technical component is performed by a technician that is billed with the NPI of the physician who provided direct supervision (in the facility and available), the audiologist can then interpret and write the report of the findings and file the claim under the audiologist's NPI with the 26 modifier. The reimbursement is the same for the TC + PC components as it is when the global code is billed; there is no reduction in payment.

52   Reduced Services
The most common audiology applications are when only one ear is tested or if not all components of a test were completed, such as not performing bone conduction as part of the comprehensive audiometry code 92557.

59   Distinct Procedure Service
This is to be used to indicate when two or more procedures not typically performed on the same date of service are appropriate to be billed due to the National Correct Coding Initiative (NCCI edits). One of the only times an audiologist would use this modifier is if not all four tests of 92540 were performed, which would be performing 1 to 3 of the following codes: 92541, 92542, 92544, or 92545. For example, if an audiologist only performed 92541 and 92542, it would be filed as 92541-59 and 92542-59. An explanation can be found here: http://www.cms.gov/Medicare/Coding/NationalCorrectCodInitEd/Downloads/modifier59.pdf.

How CPT® Codes Are Valued

Briefly, each code has three components, one of which, the Relative Value Unit for work, is listed below for many codes pertinent to audiologists. Codes are created and valued at the American Medical Association's CPT® Panel and at the RUC, the specialty society Relative Value Scale Update Committee, and are the AMA's copyrighted intellectual property. The first component is work (wRVU), which accounts for approximately 48% of the value and includes the time, technical skills, and the mental effort to perform the test. The second component, practice expense (peRVU), includes office expenses such as rent, staff, and equipment and also averages 48% of the code's value. The remainder of the value is malpractice or professional liability insurance (pliRVU) (AMA, 2016). The three RVU components are added together (wRVU + peRVU + pliRVU) and then multiplied by the Geographic Price Cost Index (GPCI) for each of the work, practice expense, and liability components (wRVU × GPCI + peRVU × GPCI + pliRVU × GPCI) which takes into account the areas where services are provided and is now the total RVU. Different parts of the country have different GPCIs as, for example, the cost of living in Manhattan is higher than in a rural area. The final component to this intricate formula is the Conversion Factor (CF) determined by Congress, which is then multiplied by the total RVU for the final calculation (Total RVU × CF), the amount that Medicare deems as the Medicare Physician Fee Schedule (MPFS), adjusted annually; many payers use this fee schedule to set their own fees. Once these values are established they are not changed unless the Centers for Medicare and Medicaid Services directs a process spawned by data mining targeting utilization, the use of screens for procedures that are performed on the same date of service, or other policies that direct code valuation.

Drilling down into the wRVU, there are three components: The preservice time (greeting the patient and getting them ready for the procedure), the intra-service time (the time for the actual procedure), and the postservice time (going over the test results, report writing, cleaning the room, etc.). These work components are critical and are primarily the reason for the decrease in reimbursement for many codes utilized by audiologists seen in recent years. Medicare screens their captured utilization data and directs their attention to when several tests are performed on the same date of service. For example, 92570 (tympanometry, acoustic reflex thresholds, and acoustic decay) became a bundled code of these separate and distinct procedures when two pre-, intra-, and postservice times were eliminated since three procedures are now performed as one procedure code with one pre-, intra-, and postservice time. This results in a decrease in reimbursement since two pre-, intra-, and postservice times are eliminated. In the last decade, these changes have been devastating to audiology and have resulted in some practices discontinuing the impacted services.

Another factor in Medicare payment impacting audiology was the transition from the non-physician work pool to work recognition, as payments were based on the more lucrative practice expense, but the offset is that as a profession, audiologists are then recognized for the necessary skills to perform the test. Most audiology CPT® codes have values as described, but the HCPCS codes do not; therefore, a third-party payer can choose to pay via the methodology they choose, which is vastly different between payers and may seem arbitrary to providers.

The Following Are the CPT® Codes and Their Work RVUs

Vestibular Function Tests

92537   Caloric vestibular test with recording, bilateral; bithermal (i.e., one warm and one cool irrigation in each ear for a total of four irrigations).
wRVU .60

92538   Monothermal (i.e., one irrigation in each ear for a total of two irrigations).
wRVU.30

92540   Basic vestibular evaluation, includes spontaneous nystagmus test with eccentric gaze fixation nystagmus, with recording, positional nystagmus test, minimum of 4 positions, with recording, optokinetic nystagmus test, bidirectional foveal and peripheral stimulation, with recording, and oscillating tracking test, with recording.
wRVU 1.50

92541   Spontaneous nystagmus test, including gaze and fixation nystagmus, with recording.
wRVU 0.40

92542   Positional nystagmus test, minimum of 4 positions, with recording.
wRVU 0.48

92544 Optokinetic nystagmus test, bidirectional, foveal, or peripheral stimulation, with recording.
wRVU 0.27

92545 Oscillating tracking test, with recording.
wRVU 0.25

92546 Sinusoidal vertical axis rotational testing.
wRVU 0.29

+92547 Use of vertical electrodes (list separately in addition to code for primary procedure).
wRVU 0.00

92548 Computerized dynamic posturography.
wRVU 0.50

Audiological Tests

92550 Tympanometry and reflex threshold measurements.
wRVU 0.35

92552 Pure tone audiometry (threshold); air only.
wRVU 0.00

92553 Air and bone.
wRVU 0.00

92555 Speech audiometry threshold.
wRVU 0.00

92556 With speech recognition.
wRVU 0.00

92557 Comprehensive audiometry threshold evaluation and speech recognition (92553 and 92556 combined).
wRVU 0.60

92558 Evoked otoacoustic emissions, screening (qualitative measurement of distortion product or transient evoked otoacoustic emissions), automated analysis.
wRVU 0.00

92567 Tympanometry (impedance testing).
wRVU 0.20

92570 Acoustic immittance testing, includes tympanometry (impedance testing),

acoustic reflex threshold testing, and acoustic reflex decay testing.
wRVU 0.55

92579 Visual reinforcement audiometry (VRA).
wRVU 0.70

92582 Conditioning play audiometry.
wRVU 0.00

92584 Electrocochleography.
wRVU 0.00

92585 Auditory evoked potentials for evoked response audiometry and/or testing of the central nervous system; comprehensive.
wRVU 0.50

92587 Distortion product evoked otoacoustic emissions; limited evaluation (to confirm the presence or absence of hearing disorder, 3 to 6 frequencies) or transient evoked otoacoustic emissions, with interpretation and report.
wRVU 0.35

92588 Comprehensive diagnostic evaluation (quantitative analysis of outer hair cell function by cochlear mapping, minimum of 12 frequencies), with interpretation and report.
wRVU 0.55

92590 Hearing aid examination and selection, monaural.
wRVU 0.00

92591 Binaural.
wRVU 0.00

92592 Hearing aid check; monaural.
wRVU 0.00

92593 Binaural.
wRVU 0.00

Evaluation and Therapeutic Services

92601 Diagnostic analysis of cochlear implant, patient younger than 7 years of age; with programming.
wRVU 2.30

92602 Subsequent reprogramming.
wRVU 1.30

92603 Diagnostic analysis of cochlear implant, age 7 years or older; with programming.
wRVU 2.25

92604 Subsequent reprogramming.
wRVU 1.25

92620 Evaluation of central auditory function, with report; initial 60 minutes.
wRVU 1.50

+92621 Each additional 15 minutes (list separately in addition to code for primary procedure).
wRVU 0.35

92625 Assessment of tinnitus (includes pitch, loudness matching, and masking).
wRVU 1.15

92626 Evaluation of auditory rehabilitation status; first hour.
wRVU 1.40

+92627 Each additional 15 minutes (list separately in addition to codes for primary procedure).
wRVU 0.33

92700 Unlisted otorhinolaryngological service or procedure.
wRVU 0.00

Cerumen Management (CPT® Code 69209 and 69210)

While it may be in the scope of practice of an audiologist in most states, Medicare does not recognize audiologists for cerumen management. Since it is a never covered Medicare service, if the patient chooses to have this performed, they may pay privately for CPT® code 69209 or 69210. A voluntary Advanced Beneficiary Notice may be offered to the Medicare patient to alert them of their financial responsibility.

Impaction is defined as "cerumen impairs exam of clinically significant portions of the external auditory canal, tympanic membrane, or middle ear condition" and "obstructive, copious cerumen that cannot be removed without magnification

and multiple instrumentations requiring physician skills" (AMA CPT® Assistant, 2016).

Specific Audiology Issues

Evaluation and Management Codes (99201-99205, New Patient, 99211-99215, Established Patient)

An area of debate is whether an audiologist may report an Evaluation and Management (E/M) code. Currently, Medicare does not recognize these codes when performed by an audiologist and as a result, other payers have followed this guidance. Audiologists employed by otolaryngologists should not report E/M codes on the same date of service as the ENT visit as those payers who may recognize an E/M code when filed by an audiologist will not likely do so when the ENT in the same office also reported an E/M service on the same date for the same patient. Check with your local payers as well as state licensure laws and be very familiar with the front section detailing the requirements of E/M codes in the CPT® codebook as well as the 1997 Medicare Documentation Guidelines for Evaluation and Management Codes.

Billing Provider Guidelines

As previously discussed, Medicare will allow a technician to perform the technical component of tests that have separate technical and professional components (e.g., ENG/VNG, sinusoidal vertical axis rotational testing, computerized dynamic posturography, limited and comprehensive otoacoustic emissions, comprehensive auditory brainstem response) when the billing/supervising physician provides general supervision. General supervision means the procedure is furnished under the physician's overall direction and control, but the physician's presence is not required during the performance of the procedure. The technical services performed by the technician are then billed under the supervising physician's NPI with modifier TC. Under general supervision, the training of the non-physician personnel who actually performs the diagnostic procedure and the maintenance of the necessary equipment and supplies are the continuing responsibility of the physician. Technicians can only perform the test and not any interpretive services.

Audiologists may also perform the test if someone else (e.g., physician, non-physician practitioner) is providing the interpretation and report. The audiologist would report the appropriate codes with modifier TC. When an audiologist only performs the interpretation and report, that test is then billed by the audiologist with modifier 26. If the same audiologist performs the test as well as completes the interpretation and report, it is reported as a global code, without any modifiers. The reimbursement is the same when the TC and PC components are filed separately as the reimbursement for filing the global codes.

The following scenarios offer how different providers may perform the test and bill Medicare as well as for those commercial payers that follow Medicare guidelines for those codes that have technical and professional components:

Scenario 1: The audiologist performs both the technical and professional components of the test (performs the test, interprets the results, and writes the report). The code, without a modifier, is billed with the audiologist's NPI.

Scenario 2: The technician performs the test under general physician supervision and the audiologist does the interpretation and writes the report. For example, if the technician performed CPT® code 92585, Auditory evoked potentials for evoked response audiometry and/or testing of the central nervous system; comprehensive, the supervising physician reports the test performed by the technician as 92585 with the TC modifier (technical component) and the audiologist interprets the test and writes the report, filing the claim as 92585 with the 26 modifier, to indicate the professional component.

Scenario 3: The technician performs the test under general physician supervision and the same physician performs the interpretation and report. The physician reports the code without a modifier.

Scenario 4: While the least likely of these scenarios, the audiologist performs the test and the physician (or non-physician provider such as a nurse practitioner, a physician's assistant, etc.) performs the interpretation and report. The audiologist reports the code with modifier TC and the physician/non-physician provider reports the code with modifier 26.

Check with your private payers for their guidelines. Most will separately credential audiologists as an independent billing provider which will keep their charges, collections, and other measures of productivity consistently aligned with the provider performing the service rather than a supervising physician.

Key Points

- Diagnostic services performed by an audiologist should be billed to Medicare by way of the providing audiologist's NPI number. In order to do so, this requires being enrolled in Medicare, having a Provider Transaction Access Number (PTAN), and a physician order based on medical necessity.
- Currently, Medicare recognizes audiologists as diagnosticians only and not as providers of treatment or therapy services such as cerumen removal, vestibular rehabilitation, and/or tinnitus management. These services can still be performed since they are in an audiologist's scope of practice as long as they are recognized by their state licensure laws, but they cannot be filed to Medicare unless a denial is necessary in order for a secondary payer to pay their portion. If a secondary payer also does not recognize these services, the patient should expect to be held responsible for payment.
- Utilize as specific a diagnostic code as possible and minimize the use of unspecified codes to decrease the chance of denials. With the ICD-10 family of codes, the increase in specificity and laterality is exponential when compared to the ICD-9s, but one transition change that should be helpful is to include any co-morbidities

(diabetes, ototoxicity and causative factors, etc. also need to be included).

- Comprehensive audiometry threshold evaluation and speech recognition (92553 and 92556 combined), 92557, one of the profession's core procedures, includes the combination of 92553 (pure tone audiometry [threshold], air, and bone) as well as 92556 (speech audiometry threshold; with speech recognition).
- Basic vestibular evaluation testing (92540) includes four component tests: spontaneous nystagmus test, including gaze and fixation, with recording (92541), positional nystagmus test, minimum of 4 positions, with recording (92542), optokinetic nystagmus test, bidirectional, foveal or peripheral stimulation, with recording (92544), and oscillating tracking test, with recording (92545). However, caloric testing may be reported with either one unit of the bithermal and bilateral caloric code (one warm, one cool, both ears), 92537, or with one unit of the monothermal code (same temperature, both ears), 92538.
- All audiology diagnostic testing codes assume bilateral testing.
- All audiological services require an interpretation and written report in the chart notes and a report to the ordering physician; diagnostic testing services should also include a printout or diagram of the results, contained within the patient's medical record.

Evaluation and Management (E/M) Codes

Evaluation and Management (E/M) codes, CPT® 99201-99205, office or other outpatient visit for a new patient and 99211-99215 for an established patient, also need to be addressed when discussing CPT® codes. An established patient is one who has been seen in the office within the last three years. Medicare does not recognize E/M codes when performed and filed by an audiologist, but other third-party payers may. If any audiologist chooses to utilize this code family, caution is urged as they are time and medical complexity based and also involve a Review of Systems (ROS). The author urges that any audiologist who is contemplating using E/M codes read the front section of the CPT® codebook and the Centers for Medicare and Medicaid Services 1997 Documentation Guidelines for Evaluation and Management Services. It is also recommended that you obtain written guidance from your payers as some of the major commercial payers disallow audiologists from filing claims for E/M codes. It would be wise for the audiologist to log in the time they started the E/M service and the time it ended in their chart documentation and not file a claim strictly based on the time of the code as this will likely lead to potential upcoding, audits, and payback of payments. Audiologists in otolaryngology offices will likely have difficulty with these codes if the otolaryngologist also files them for the same date of service as the audiologist's E/M code will not be paid, but the physician's will. Another word of caution is that of the E/M codes, only 99201, 99202, 99211, and 99212 are suggested for utilization by audiologists, once you have payer confirmation when an audiologist performs these services.

Healthcare Common Procedure Coding System II (HCPCS II) Codes

The Healthcare Common Procedure Coding System Level II (HCPCS) V codes are for hearing and vision services. The hearing services codes (V5000-V5299) include a few procedures, but the remainder of these codes is for the type, style, and technology of the hearing aid and the professional services associated with those styles or technology. The HCPCS II L codes are for "Orthotic/Prosthetic Procedures," which include the cochlear implant and auditory osseo-integrated devices. Typically the physician bills for the surgical code; however, most often the device is supplied and billed by the facility where the surgical implantation occurs. The L codes are utilized by audiologists for cochlear implant and osseo-integrated devices, repairs, and/or supplies. The

HCPCS II codes also include an S code as an option for audiometry for an HAE to determine the level and degree of hearing loss (S0618) and for deluxe item patient aware, in addition to basic code (S1001) for hearing aid upgrades beyond the patient's benefit, if either is recognized by the payer. If not recognized by the payer, the patient needs to be counseled that when they receive their Explanation of Benefits (EOB) that their benefit is typically for covered services and upgrades are non-covered services that are not always specified on the EOB but are the patient's responsibility. S codes are usually recognized by some private payers such as Blue Cross Blue Shield.

L Codes for Cochlear Implants and Osseo-Integrated Devices

L7510   Repair of prosthetic device, repair or replace minor parts

L7520   Repair prosthetic device, labor component, per 15 minutes

L8614   Cochlear device, includes all internal and external components

L8615   Headset/headpiece for use with cochlear implant device, replacement

L8616   Microphone for use with cochlear implant device, replacement

L8617   Transmitting coil for use with cochlear implant device, replacement

L8618   Transmitter cable for use with cochlear implant device, replacement

L8619   Cochlear implant, external speech processor and controller, integrated system, replacement

L8621   Zinc air battery for use with cochlear implant device and auditory osseo-integrated sound processors, replacement, each

L8622   Alkaline battery for use with cochlear implant device, any size, replacement, each

L8623   Lithium ion battery for use with cochlear implant device speech processor, other than ear level, replacement, each

L8624   Lithium ion battery for use with cochlear implant device speech processor, ear level, replacement, each

L8627   Cochlear implant, external speech processor, component, replacement

L8628   Cochlear implant, external controller component, replacement

L8629   Transmitting coil and cable, integrated, for use with cochlear implant device, replacement

L8690   Auditory osseo-integrated device, includes all internal and external components

L8691   Auditory osseo-integrated device, external sound processor, replacement

L8692   Auditory osseo-integrated device, external sound processor, used without osseointegration, body worn, includes headband or other means of external attachment

L8693   Auditory osseo-integrated device abutment, any length, replacement only

L9900   Orthotic and prosthetic supply, accessory, and/or service component of another HCPCS "L" code

V Codes for Hearing Aid Related Services

V5008   Hearing screening

V5010   Assessment for hearing aid

V5011   Fitting/orientation/checking of hearing aid

V5014   Repair/modification of a hearing aid

V5020   Conformity evaluation

V5030   Hearing aid, monaural, body worn, air conduction

V5040   Hearing aid, monaural, body worn, bone conduction

V5050   Hearing aid, monaural, in the ear

V5060   Hearing aid, monaural, behind the ear

V5070 Glasses, air conduction

V5080 Glasses, bone conduction

V5090 Dispensing fee, unspecified hearing aid

V5095 Semi-implantable middle ear hearing prosthesis

V5100 Hearing aid, bilateral, body worn

V5110 Dispensing fee, bilateral

V5120 Binaural, body

V5130 Binaural, in the ear

V5140 Binaural, behind the ear

V5150 Binaural, glasses

V5160 Dispensing fee, binaural

V5170 Hearing aid, CROS, in the ear

V5180 Hearing aid, CROS, behind the ear

V5190 Hearing aid, CROS, glasses

V5200 Dispensing fee, CROS

V5210 Hearing aid, BICROS, in the ear

V5220 Hearing aid, BICROS, behind the ear

V5230 Hearing aid, BICROS, glasses

V5240 Dispensing fee, BICROS

V5241 Dispensing fee, monaural hearing aid, any type

V5242 Hearing aid, analog, monaural CIC (completely in the ear canal)

V5243 Hearing aid, analog, monaural, ITC (in the canal)

V5244 Hearing aid, digitally programmable analog, monaural, CIC

V5245 Hearing aid, digitally programmable analog, monaural, ITC

V5246 Hearing aid, digitally programmable analog, monaural, ITE (in the ear)

V5247 Hearing aid, digitally programmable analog, monaural, BTE (behind the ear)

V5248 Hearing aid, analog, binaural, CIC

V5249 Hearing aid, analog, binaural, ITC

V5250 Hearing aid, digitally programmable analog, binaural, CIC

V5251 Hearing aid, digitally programmable analog, binaural, ITC

V5252 Hearing aid, digitally programmable, binaural, ITE

V5253 Hearing aid, digitally programmable, binaural, BTE

V5254 Hearing aid, digital, monaural, CIC

V5255 Hearing aid, digital, monaural, ITC

V5256 Hearing aid, digital, monaural, ITE

V5257 Hearing aid, digital, monaural, BTE

V5258 Hearing aid, digital, binaural, CIC

V5259 Hearing aid, digital, binaural, ITC

V5260 Hearing aid, digital, binaural, ITE

V5261 Hearing aid, digital, binaural, BTE

V5262 Hearing aid, disposable, any type, monaural

V5263 Hearing aid, disposable, any type, binaural

V5264 Ear mold/insert, not disposable, any type

V5265 Ear mold/insert, disposable, any type

V5266 Battery for use in hearing device

V5267 Hearing aid or assistive listening device/supplies/accessories, not otherwise specified

V5268 Assistive listening device, telephone amplifier, any type

V5269 Assistive listening device, alerting, any type

V5270 Assistive listening device, television amplifier, any type

V5271 Assistive listening device, television caption decoder

V5272 Assistive listening device, TDD

V5273 Assistive listening device, for use with cochlear implant

V5274 Assistive listening device, not otherwise specified

V5275 Ear impression, each

V5281 Assistive listening device, personal FM/DM system, monaural (1 receiver, transmitter, microphone), any type

V5282 Assistive listening device, personal FM/DM system, binaural (2 receivers, transmitter, microphone), any type

V5283 Assistive listening device, personal FM/DM neck, loop induction receiver

V5284 Assistive listening device, personal FM/DM, ear level receiver

V5285 Assistive listening device, personal FM/DM, direct audio input

V5286 Assistive listening device, personal blue tooth FM/DM receiver

V5287 Assistive listening device, personal FM/DM receiver, not otherwise specified

V5288 Assistive listening device, personal FM/DM transmitter assistive listening device

V5289 Assistive listening device, personal FM/DM adapter/boot coupling device for receiver, any type

V5290 Assistive listening device, transmitter microphone, any type

V5298 Hearing aid, not otherwise classified

V5299 Hearing service, miscellaneous

Key ICD-10-CM Codes

After several delays, the ICD-10-CM and ICD-10-PCS disease codes were transitioned in October 2015, the first coding change in the United States in 30 years. Many ICD-10-CMs are included below as these are the codes utilized by private practice or otolaryngology office audiologists among other non-inpatient settings. Those in a hospital setting will use ICD-10-PCS, a different coding system. In the ICD-10-CM coding system, the most frequent disease codes utilized by audiologists fall under several sections: Disorders of vestibular function (H81.0-H81.93), vertiginous syndromes in diseases classified elsewhere (H82.1-H82.9), other diseases of the inner ear (H83.0-H83.9), and the hearing loss codes, H83.3-H93.9. These are to be selected based on the outcome of the test results or the reason for the tests, which may also include signs or symptoms and must be a part of the documentation in the patient's medical record. The more specific the code, the lesser chance for denial; therefore, it is preferred that the unspecified codes not be utilized. With ICD-10s, it is not just about the balance disorder and/or the hearing loss, but also noting and coding for comorbidities which impact hearing and balance such as dizziness, renal disease, ototoxicity, and the causative offender, to name just a few, if applicable. These should be included in the audiologist's chart notes, regardless of work setting.

There are several considerations within ICD-10s that are different from the previous coding (ICD-9) system:

- Unilateral hearing loss codes suggest normal or near normal hearing thresholds in the opposite ear when the description includes "with unrestricted hearing on the contralateral side"
- There is no distinction between sensory hearing loss or neural hearing loss; they are combined as sensorineural hearing loss
- The middle ear hearing loss codes were classified by their location in the ear (e.g., tympanic membrane, middle ear), but are not specified as such in the ICD-10-CM system, but combined as conductive hearing loss
- Effective October 1, 2016, several new diagnoses codes became effective including those for conductive, sensorineural, and mixed hearing losses, restricted ear(s), to allow different types of hearing loss

in different ears to be specifically coded for that ear, which was not as specific in the ICD-9 system. Each ear will require a restricted code for that specific ear for a total of two ICD-10-CM codes for each procedure, one code for the right ear and one for the left. For example, if a patient had a sensorineural hearing loss in the right ear and a conductive hearing loss in the left, you would code H90.A21 for the right ear and H90.A12 for the left, for the procedure(s) performed. Otherwise, for one ear that is normal or near normal, the unrestricted code applies and is the only one needed, such as when a patient has a conductive hearing loss in the right ear and normal or near normal hearing acuity in the left, which for this example is H90.11.

- Also effective October 1, 2016, codes for pulsatile tinnitus joined the existing tinnitus codes of H93.11-H93.19. Pulsatile tinnitus, right ear is H93.A1, pulsatile tinnitus, left ear is H93.A2, and pulsatile tinnitus, bilateral is H93.A3.

In the ICD-10-CM coding system, typically laterality is addressed with the following ear indicators as the last character of a code, with some exceptions:

- 1 = right ear
- 2 = left ear
- 3 = bilateral
- 0 or 9 = unspecified

Examples of commonly used code families are

H61.2-H61.23	Impacted cerumen
H81.0-H81.09	Meniere's disease
H81.1-H81.13	Benign paroxysmal vertigo
H81.2-H81.23	Vestibular neuronitis
H83.0-H83.09	Labyrinthitis
H83.3-H83.3X9-	Noise effects on inner ear
H91.2-H91.23	Sudden idiopathic hearing loss

H93.21-H93.219	Auditory recruitment
H93.22-H93.229	Diplacusis
H93.23-H93.239	Hyperacusis
H93.25	Central auditory processing disorder
H93.8-H93.299	Other abnormal auditory perceptions
H93.1-H93.19	Tinnitus
H93.24-H93.249	Temporary auditory threshold shift
H90.2	Conductive hearing loss, unspecified
H90.11	Conductive hearing loss, unilateral, right ear, with unrestricted hearing on the contralateral side
H90.0	Conductive hearing loss, bilateral
H90.5	Unspecified sensorineural hearing loss
H90.41	Sensorineural hearing loss, unilateral, right ear, with unrestricted hearing on the contralateral side
H90.3	Sensorineural hearing loss, bilateral
H90.8	Mixed conductive and sensorineural hearing loss, unspecified
H90.71	Mixed conductive and sensorineural hearing loss, unilateral, right ear, with unrestricted hearing on the contralateral side
H90.6	Mixed conductive and sensorineural hearing loss, bilateral
H91.90	Unspecified hearing loss, unspecified ear
R42	Dizziness and giddiness

Non-Hearing Loss ICD-10 Codes for Consideration

The following codes are offered as secondary, third, fourth, and so on code considerations with a hearing loss code as the primary for those with ototoxicity (H90.0-H90.09), infections, cancer, and so on, and used in addition to the applicable T code indicating the biologic given that may have contributed to the hearing loss associated with ototoxicity and/or any of these diseases or systemic problems. This should be described in the patient's chart notes.

A40-A49.9	Bacterial infection
B50-B54	Malaria related codes
B95-B95.8	Streptococcus, staphylococcus, enterococcus, MRSA infection
C00-C72.59	Malignant neoplasms infection
D00-D49.6	Neoplasms
F80.1	Expressive language disorder
F80.4	Speech delay due to hearing loss
F81.89	Other developmental disorders of scholastic skills
Q16-Q17.4	Congenital malformations of the ear causing hearing impairment
R62.0	Delayed milestones in childhood, late talker
R94.120	Abnormal auditory function study
R94.121	Abnormal vestibular function study
R94.122	Abnormal results of other function studies of ear and other special sense
T36.3-T59	Poisoning by macrolides, aminoglycosides, salicylates, aspirin, non-steroidal anti-inflammatory drugs, methadone, anti-neoplastic and immunosuppressive drugs, vasodilators, loop diuretics, organic solvents (benzene, organic solvents, lead, mercury, other metals, arsenic, manganese, carbon monoxide, other gases/fumes/vapors)
T70.0XXA-T70.0XXS	Otic barotrauma
Z01.10-Z97.4	These codes may be used as secondary or other subsequent codes for the following: encounter for examination and hearing without abnormal findings, encounter for examination and hearing with abnormal findings, failed hearing screening, hearing conservation and treatment, management of implanted device, bone conduction device, cochlear device, fitting/adjustment of hearing aid, occupational exposure to noise, person consulting for explanation of examination or test findings, malingerer, family history of ear disorders, cochlear implant status, myringotomy tube status, and presence of other otological and audiological implants.

Most payers are *not* recognizing these codes are primary diagnosis codes. In that scenario, it is best to code by the reason for the test, their signs and symptoms, and/or the outcome of the test results and use these codes as secondary or beyond codes, thinking of them as supplemental to the primary diagnosis.

Now that you have a basic foundation of the codes available for audiologists, the next logical step is to understand Medicare requirements and regulations pertaining to audiologic services in order for correct and proper utilization when billed to the largest and most stringent payer as well as to all third-party payers.

References

American Medical Association. (2016) *CPT® Assistant*. 26, 1, 7–8.

American Medical Association. (2016). Retrieved on April 1, 2016 from http://www.ama-assn.org/ama/pub/physician -resources/solutions-managing-your-practice/coding

-billing-insurance/medicare/the-resource-based-relative-value-scale/overview-of-rbrvs.page?

Centers for Medicare and Medicaid Services. (1997). 1997 Documentation Guidelines for Evaluation and Management Codes. Retrieved on April 1, 2016 from https://www.cms.gov/Outreach-and-Education/Medicare-Learning-Network-MLN/MLNEdWebGuide/Downloads/97Docguidelines.pdf.

Centers for Medicare and Medicaid Services. (2002). Program Memorandum Intermediaries /Carriers Transmittal AB-02-080. Retrieved on October 25, 2015 from https://www.cms.gov/Regulations-and-Guidance/Guidance/Transmittals/downloads/AB02080.pdf.

National Correct Coding Initiative (NCCI) (2015). Modifier 59 article. Retrieved on September 12, 2016 from https://www.cms.gov/Medicare/Coding/NationalCorrectCodInitEd/Downloads/modifier59.pdf.

Office of the Inspector General. (2014). Retrieved on April 1, 2016 at http://oig.hhs.gov/fraud/enforcement/cmp/cmp-ae.asp.

CHAPTER 2

Introduction to Medicare

Debra Abel

Medicare is the largest payer and is also the payer with the most stringent rules that apply to enrolled providers. Because of the profession's Medicare status known as "other diagnostic services" defined by Social Security Act §1861(s)(3), audiologists must enroll in Medicare unless all diagnostic audiology services are provided to each patient at no charge. Physicians are allowed to opt out of Medicare which includes otolaryngologists (ENTs), but audiologists are *not*. In an otolaryngology office with audiologist employees, this could be problematic if an ENT chooses to opt out of Medicare and the enrolled practice audiologist cannot, especially when considering the ENTs are their likeliest source for orders and referrals of Medicare beneficiaries. It is imperative for every practice manager and owner to read sections 80 and 80.3 of Chapter 15, Covered Medical and Other Health Services, in the Medicare Benefits Policy Manual, most of which is included in this chapter, addressing the definition of a qualified audiologist, audiology services, physician orders, coverage, individuals who furnish audiology tests, documentation, treatment, and opting out. Another chapter of interest to audiologists is Chapter 16, General Exclusions from Coverage (https://www.cms.gov/Regulations-and -Guidance/Guidance/Manuals/Downloads/bp 102c16.pdf).

Medicare serves as the benchmark for many health care providers due to the imposed requirements, the most defined regulations applicable to audiologists; commercial payers may follow the same guidelines or create their own less stringent guidelines. Medicare tracks this coding information and policies are created in response, especially when professional trends may occur (e.g., a significant increase in utilization of a procedure over several years) and is what led to the 2012 revised descriptions of the otoacoustic emissions codes for CPT® codes 92587 and 92588. It also required bundling of procedures performed on the same date of service, thereby reducing the reimbursement due to the elimination of pre-, intra-, and post-service times that are included within the code's valuation as seen in 2010 with the vestibular code bundle 92540. Additionally, Medicare tracks what is known as outliers, those providers who bill differently than their collegial counterparts for the same services, which may trigger an audit.

Medicare requirements are the foundation of the regulations which impact performing and billing Medicare diagnostic audiology procedures. The Centers for Medicare and Medicaid Services (CMS) Program Memorandum AB-02-080 states "diagnostic testing, including hearing and balance assessment services, performed by a qualified audiologist is paid for as 'other diagnostic tests' under §1861 (s)(3) of the Social Security Act (the Act) when a physician orders testing to obtain information as part of his/her diagnostic evaluation or to determine the appropriate medical or surgical treatment of a hearing deficit or related medical problem" (CMS, 2002). This is the fundamental reason why Medicare recognizes audiologists only for diagnostic testing procedures and why a physician order is required. It would literally take an act of Congress to change these requirements.

Diagnostic audiologic services provided under the "other diagnostic test" category in section 1861(s)(3) of the Social Security Act are not to be billed as "incident to" services to Medicare. In 2008, the CMS issued Transmittal 84, which required all audiologists to bill services supplied to Medicare Part B beneficiaries under their own National Provider Identifier (NPI) and not by way of the NPI of a physician. Unfortunately, this practice of billing audiology services performed by an audiologist and billed by an otolaryngologist continues and if discovered, Medicare will likely seek repayments as well as penalties and interest.

At the time of publication, Medicare continues to recognize audiologists only as diagnosticians, not providers of treatment of hearing and balance disorders such as the rehabilitation of hearing loss, tinnitus management, and management of those experiencing imbalance disorders. Although more restrictive in scope than state licensure laws which define a provider's scope of practice allowing diagnosis and treatment, some payers do recognize and reimburse for all professional services that audiologists are licensed to provide. It behooves a practice to be aware of the differences in requirements for audiological services among payers. It is also important to remember that as long as it is not contractually excluded, patients should expect to pay for items and services not covered by their third-party payers which includes Medicare.

Medicare Benefits Policy Manual Chapter 15: The Critical Foundation for Billing Audiologic Services

The following excerpts are the essential portions of section 80.3 of Chapter 15 of the Medicare Benefits Policy manual to provide the understanding of what Medicare requirements are and the necessity of following this guidance in order to be compliant with Medicare policies.

Chapter 15 of the Medicare Benefits Policy Manual, Section 80.3

80.3.1 Definition of Qualified Audiologist

This section defines what requirements an audiologist must meet in order to provide diagnostic services to Medicare.

"Audiological tests require the skills of an audiologist and shall be furnished by qualified audiologists, or, in States where it is allowed by State and local laws, by a physician or Non-physician practitioner. Medicare is not authorized to pay for these services when performed by audiological aides, assistants, technicians, or others who do not meet the qualifications below. In cases where it is not clear, the Medicare contractor shall determine whether a service is an audiological service that requires the skills of an audiologist and whether the qualifications for an audiologist have been met.

Section 1861(ll)(3) of the Act provides that a qualified audiologist is an individual with a master's or doctoral degree in audiology. Therefore, a Doctor of Audiology (AuD) 4th year student with a provisional license from a State does not qualify unless he or she also holds a master's or doctoral degree in audiology. In addition, a qualified audiologist is an individual who:

- Is licensed as an audiologist by the State in which the individual furnishes such services, or
- In the case of an individual who furnishes services in a State which does not license audiologists has:
  - Successfully completed 350 clock hours of supervised clinical practicum (or is in the process of accumulating such supervised clinical experience),
  - Performed not less than 9 months of supervised full-time audiology services after obtaining a master's or doctoral degree in audiology or a related field, and
  - Successfully completed a national examination in audiology approved by the Secretary.

If it is necessary to determine whether a particular audiologist is qualified under the above definition, the carrier should check references. Carriers in States that have statutory licensure or certification should secure from the appropriate State agency a current listing of audiologists holding the required credentials. Additional references for determining an audiologist's professional qualifications are the national directory published annually by the American Speech-Language-Hearing Association and records and directories, which may be available from the State Licensing Authority" (CMS, 2015).

Benefits Under Medicare

- "Hearing and balance assessment services are generally covered as 'other diagnostic tests' under section 1861(s)(3) of the Social Security Act. Hearing and balance assessment services furnished to an outpatient of a hospital are covered as 'diagnostic services' under section 1861(s)(2)(C).
- As defined in the Social Security Act, section 1861(ll)(3), the term 'audiology services' specifically means such hearing and balance assessment services furnished by a qualified audiologist as the audiologist is legally authorized to perform under State law (or the State regulatory mechanism provided by State law), as would otherwise be covered if furnished by a physician" (CMS 2015).

Orders

- "Audiology tests are covered as 'other diagnostic tests' under section 1861(s)(3) or 1861(s)(2)(C) of the Act in the physician's office or hospital outpatient settings, respectively, when a physician (or an NPP, as applicable) orders such testing for the purpose of obtaining information necessary for the physician's diagnostic medical evaluation or to determine the appropriate medical or surgical treatment of a hearing deficit or related medical problem. See section 80.6 of this chapter for policies regarding the ordering of diagnostic tests.
- If a beneficiary undergoes diagnostic testing performed by an audiologist without a physician order, the tests are not covered even if the audiologist discovers a pathologic condition.
- When a qualified physician orders a qualified technician (see definition in subsection D of this section) to furnish an appropriate audiology service, that order must specify which test is to be furnished by the technician under the direct supervision of a physician. Only that test may be provided on that order by the technician.
- When the qualified physician or NPP orders diagnostic audiology services furnished by an audiologist without naming specific tests, the audiologist may select the appropriate battery of tests" (CMS, 2015).

Coverage and Payment for Medicare Audiology Diagnostic Services

"Coverage and, therefore, payment for audiological diagnostic tests is determined by the reason the tests were performed, rather than by the diagnosis or the patient's condition. Under any Medicare payment system, payment for audiological diagnostic tests is not allowed by virtue of their exclusion from coverage in section 1862(a)(7) of the Social Security Act when:

- The type and severity of the current hearing, tinnitus, or balance status needed to determine the appropriate medical or surgical treatment is known to the physician before the test; or
- The test was ordered for the specific purpose of fitting or modifying a hearing aid.

Payment of audiological diagnostic tests is allowed for other reasons and is not limited, for example, by:

- Any information resulting from the test, for example:
- Confirmation of a prior diagnosis;
- Post-evaluation diagnoses; or
- Treatment provided after diagnosis, including hearing aids, or
- The type of evaluation or treatment the physician anticipates before the diagnostic test; or
- Timing of reevaluation. Reevaluation is appropriate at a schedule dictated by the ordering physician when the information provided by the diagnostic test is required, for example, to determine changes in hearing, to evaluate the appropriate medical or surgical treatment, or to evaluate the results of treatment. For example, reevaluation may be appropriate, even when the evaluation was recent, in cases where the hearing loss, balance, or tinnitus may be progressive or fluctuating, the patient or caregiver complains of new symptoms, or treatment (such as medication or surgery) may have changed the patient's audiological condition with or without awareness by the patient.

Reasons for Ordering Audiologic Tests

Examples of appropriate reasons for ordering audiological diagnostic tests that could be covered include, but are not limited to:

- Evaluation of suspected change in hearing, tinnitus, or balance;
- Evaluation of the cause of disorders of hearing, tinnitus, or balance;
- Determination of the effect of medication, surgery, or other treatment;
- Reevaluation to follow-up changes in hearing, tinnitus, or balance that may be caused by established diagnoses that place the patient at probable risk for a change in status including, but not limited to: otosclerosis, atelectatic tympanic membrane, tympanosclerosis, cholesteatoma, resolving middle ear

infection, Meniére's disease, sudden idiopathic sensorineural hearing loss, autoimmune inner ear disease, acoustic neuroma, demyelinating diseases, ototoxicity secondary to medications, or genetic vascular and viral conditions;
- Failure of a screening test (although the screening test is not covered);
- Diagnostic analysis of cochlear or brainstem implant and programming; and
- Audiology diagnostic tests before and periodically after implantation of auditory prosthetic devices.

If a physician refers a beneficiary to an audiologist for testing related to signs or symptoms associated with hearing loss, balance disorder, tinnitus, ear disease, or ear injury, the audiologist's diagnostic testing services should be covered even if the only outcome is the prescription of a hearing aid" (CMS, 2015).

Individuals Who Furnish Audiology Services

Audiologists

Audiologists are defined by the Social Security Act, section 1861(ll)(3) as:

"Audiological tests require the skills of an audiologist and shall be furnished by qualified audiologists, or, in States where it is allowed by State and local laws, by a physician or Non-physician practitioner.

Medicare is not authorized to pay for these services when performed by audiological aides, assistants, technicians, or others who do not meet the qualifications below. In cases where it is not clear, the Medicare contractor shall determine whether a service is an audiological service that requires the skills of an audiologist and whether the qualifications for an audiologist have been met.

Section 1861(ll)(3) of the Act provides that a qualified audiologist is an individual with a master's or doctoral degree in audiology. Therefore, a Doctor of Audiology (AuD) 4th year student with a provisional license from a State does not qualify unless he or she also holds a master's or doctoral degree in audiology. In addition, a qualified audiologist is an individual who:

- Is licensed as an audiologist by the State in which the individual furnishes such services, or
- In the case of an individual who furnishes services in a State which does not license audiologists has:
  - ○ Successfully completed 350 clock hours of supervised clinical practicum (or is in the process of accumulating such supervised clinical experience),
  - ○ Performed not less than 9 months of supervised full-time audiology services after obtaining a master's or doctoral degree in audiology or a related field, and
  - ○ Successfully completed a national examination in audiology approved by the Secretary.

Qualified Technicians or Other Qualified Staff

"The qualifications for technicians vary locally and may also depend on the type of test, the patient, and the level of participation of the physician who is directly supervising the test. Therefore, an individual must meet qualifications appropriate to the service furnished as determined by the contractor to whom the claim is billed. If it is necessary to determine whether the individual who furnished the labor for appropriate audiology services is qualified, contractors may request verification of any relevant education and training that has been completed by the technician, which shall be available in the records of the clinic or facility.

Depending on the qualifications determined by the contractor, individuals who are also hearing instrument specialists, students of audiology, or other health care professionals may furnish the labor for appropriate audiology services under direct physician when these services are billed by physicians or hospital outpatient departments" (CMS, 2015).

Documentation for Audiology Services

1. Documentation for orders (reasons for tests). "The reason for the test should be documented either on the order, on the audiological evaluation report, or in the patient's medical record. (See subsection C of this section concerning reasons for tests.)
2. Documenting skilled services. When the medical record is subject to medical review, it is necessary that the record contains sufficient information so that the contractor may determine that the service qualifies for payment. For example, documentation should indicate that the test was ordered, that the reason for the test results in coverage, and that the test was furnished to the patient by a qualified individual.

Records that support the appropriate provision of an audiological diagnostic test shall be made available to the contractor on request" (CMS, 2015).

Audiological Treatment

"There is no provision in the law for Medicare to pay audiologists for therapeutic services.

For example, vestibular treatment, auditory rehabilitation treatment, auditory processing treatment, and canalith repositioning, while they are generally within the scope of practice of audiologists, are not those hearing and balance assessment services that are defined as audiology services in 1861(ll)(3) of the Social Security Act and, therefore, shall not be billed by audiologists to Medicare. Services for the purpose of hearing aid evaluation and fitting are not covered regardless of how they are billed.

Services identified as "always" therapy in Pub. 100-04, chapter 5, section 20 may not be billed by hospitals, physicians, NPPs, or audiologists when provided by audiologists. (See also Pub. 100-04, chapter 12, section 30.3.) Treatment related to hearing may be covered under the speech-language pathology benefit when the services are provided by speech-language pathologists. Treatment related to balance (e.g., services described by "always therapy" codes 97001-97004, 97110, 97112, 97116, and 97750) may be covered under the physical therapy or occupational therapy benefit when the services are provided by therapists or their assistants, where appropriate. Covered therapy services incident to a physician's service must conform to policies in sections 60, 220, and 230 of this chapter. Audiological treatment provided under the benefits for physical therapy and speech-language pathology services may also be personally provided and billed by physicians and NPPs when the services are within their scope of practice and consistent with State and local laws.

For example, aural rehabilitation and signed communication training may be payable according to the benefit for speech-language pathology services or as speech-language pathology services incident to a physician's or NPP's service. Treatment for balance disorders may be payable according to the benefit for physical therapy services or as a physical therapy service incident to the services of a physician or NPP. See the policies in this chapter, sections 220 and 230, for details" (CMS, 2015).

Assignment

"Nonhospital entities billing for the audiologist's services may accept assignment under the usual procedure or, if not accepting assignment, may charge the patient and submit a nonassigned claim on their behalf" (CMS, 2015).

Opt Out and Mandatory Claims Submissions

"The opt out law does not define 'physician' or 'practitioner' to include audiologists; therefore, they may not opt out of Medicare and provide services under private contracts.

See section 40.4 of this chapter for details. When a physician or supplier furnishes a service that is covered by Medicare, then it is subject to the mandatory claim submission provisions of section 1848(g)(4) of the Social Security Act. Therefore, if an audiologist charges or attempts to charge a beneficiary any remuneration for a service that is covered by Medicare, then the audiologist must submit a claim to Medicare" (CMS, 2015).

Non-Audiology Services Furnished by Audiologists

"Audiologists may be qualified to furnish all or part of some diagnostic tests or treatments that are not defined as audiology services under the Medicare Physician Fee Service (MPFS), such as non-auditory evoked potentials or cerumen removal. Audiologists may not bill Medicare for services that are not audiology services according to Medicare's definition (see list at: www.cms .gov/therapyservices). However, the labor for the Technical Component (TC) of certain other diagnostic tests or treatment services may qualify to be billed when furnished by audiologists under physician supervision when all the appropriate policies are followed.

When furnishing services that are not on the Medicare list of audiology services, the audiologist may or may not be working within the scope of practice of an audiologist according to State law. The audiologist furnishing the service must have the qualifications that are ordinarily required of any person providing that service. Consult the following policies for details:

- Policies for physical therapy, occupational therapy, and speech-language pathology services are in sections 220 and 230 of this chapter and in Pub. 100-04, chapter 5, sections 10 and 20.
- Policies for services furnished incident to physicans' services in the physician's office are in section 60 of this chapter.
- Policies for therapeutic services furnished incident to physicians' services in the hospital outpatient setting are in chapter 6, section 20.5, of this manual.
- Policies for diagnostic tests in the physician's office are in section 80 of this chapter.
- Policies for diagnostic tests furnished in the hospital outpatient setting are in chapter 6, section 20.4, of this manual.

Therapeutic or treatment services that are not audiology services and are not "always" therapy (according to the policy in Pub.100-04, chapter 5, section 20) and are furnished by audiologists may be billed incident to the services of a physician when all other appropriate requirements are met.

In addition, the TC or facility services for diagnostic tests that are not audiology services may be billed by physicians or hospital outpatient departments when provided by qualified personnel (who may be audiologists), and physicians and hospital outpatient departments may bill for these diagnostic tests when provided by those qualified personnel under the specified level of physician supervision for the diagnostic test" (CMS, 2015).

Requirements for Ordering and Following Orders for Diagnostic Tests

Section 80.6.1 of Chapter 15, has the requirements for ordering and following orders for diagnostic tests:

"A diagnostic test includes all diagnostic x-ray tests, all diagnostic laboratory tests, and other diagnostic tests furnished to a beneficiary.

Treating Physician

A "treating physician" is a physician, as defined in §1861(r) of the Social Security Act (the Act), who furnishes a consultation or treats a beneficiary for a specific medical problem, and who uses the results of a diagnostic test in the management of the beneficiary's specific medical problem.

A radiologist performing a therapeutic interventional procedure is considered a treating physician. A radiologist performing a diagnostic interventional or diagnostic procedure is not considered a treating physician.

Treating Practitioner

A "treating practitioner" is a nurse practitioner, clinical nurse specialist, or physician assistant, as defined in §1861(s)(2)(K) of the Act, who fur-

nishes, pursuant to State law, a consultation or treats a beneficiary for a specific medical problem, and who uses the result of a diagnostic test in the management of the beneficiary's specific medical problem.

Testing Facility

A "testing facility" is a Medicare provider or supplier that furnishes diagnostic tests. A testing facility may include a physician or a group of physicians (e.g., radiologist, pathologist), a laboratory, or an independent diagnostic testing facility (IDTF).

Order

An "order" is a communication from the treating physician/practitioner requesting that a diagnostic test be performed for a beneficiary. The order may conditionally request an additional diagnostic test for a particular beneficiary if the result of the initial diagnostic test ordered yields to a certain value determined by the treating physician/practitioner (e.g., if test X is negative, then perform test Y). An order may be delivered via the following forms of communication:

- A written document signed by the treating physician/practitioner, which is hand-delivered, mailed, or faxed to the testing facility; NOTE: No signature is required on orders for clinical diagnostic tests paid on the basis of the clinical laboratory fee schedule, the physician fee schedule, or for physician pathology services;
- A telephone call by the treating physician/practitioner or his/her office to the testing facility; and
- An electronic mail by the treating physician/practitioner or his/her office to the testing facility.

If the order is communicated via telephone, both the treating physician/practitioner or his/her office, and the testing facility must document the telephone call in their respective copies of the beneficiary's medical records. While a physician order is not required to be signed, the physician must clearly document, in the medical record, his or her intent that the test be performed" (CMS, 2015).

In the CMS Medlearn document, SE 1305, those providers who may order tests are listed below, but is contingent on their individual state licensure laws. To avoid a claim denial, offices will want to ensure that their referring providers are enrolled in the Medicare Provider Enrollment, Chain, Ownership System or the claim will be denied and the patient will not be responsible for payment.

- Physician Assistants,
- Clinical Nurse Specialists,
- Nurse Practitioners,
- Clinical Psychologists,
- Interns, Residents, and Fellows,
- Certified Nurse Midwives, and
- Clinical Social Workers.

Physicians (doctor of medicine or osteopathy, doctor of dental medicine, doctor of dental surgery, doctor of podiatric medicine, doctor of optometry, optometrists may only order and refer DMEPOS products/services and laboratory and X-ray services payable under Medicare Part B" (CMS, 2015) furnished by audiologists under physician supervision when all the appropriate policies are followed.

"Incident to" Billing

In 2008, the Centers for Medicare and Medicaid Services (CMS) issued Transmittal 84, which required all audiologists to bill services supplied to Medicare Part B beneficiaries under their own National Provider Identifier (NPI) and not via the NPI of a physician. This was a sentinel moment for audiology as historically, many otolaryngologists filed Medicare claims with their NPI for audiology services. One reason for this practice may be that non-physician providers such as nurse practitioners, physician assistants, and so on are paid at 10% less of the Medicare Physician Fee Schedule. Audiologists have historically been paid at the

same rate as physicians by way of the Medicare Physician Fee Schedule and, of course, there are other possibilities that may have resulted in this faulty and incorrect practice. Unfortunately, this practice of billing audiology services performed by an audiologist and billed by an otolaryngologist continues and, if discovered, Medicare will likely seek repayments as well as penalties and interest. If there is any doubt, in 2014, an otolaryngology/audiology practice in Texas reached a $200,630 settlement for "allegations that for nearly three years the practice improperly submitted claims to Medicare and Texas Medicaid for hearing assessment services performed by unqualified technicians" (OIG, 2014). This was for "incident to" billing and illustrates that these scenarios are not being ignored.

As noted earlier, diagnostic audiology services without a technical component are never to be billed "incident to," including CPT® code 92557, basic comprehensive audiometry. These diagnostic audiology services reside in the "other diagnostic test" Medicare category and as such, are excluded from the "incident to" requirements. Providers need to check with their Medicare Administrative Contractor (MAC) for guidance on the recognition and use of automated audiometry, CPT® codes 0208T, 0209T, 0210T, 0211T, and 0212T, if this method of testing is utilized in one's office as most MACs want these services provided by an audiologist, physician, or non-physician provider.

Technicians and Medicare

If an otolaryngology practice employs a technician, Medicare allows them to only perform the technical component of these CPT® codes:

- 92537-92546, 92548 (vestibular codes)
- 92585 auditory evoked potential, comprehensive and
- 92587 (limited) and 92588 (comprehensive) otoacoustic emissions which have a technical (TC) and professional component (-26), with the physician's direct supervision. Those services are then filed via the physician's National Provider Identifier (NPI) with the TC modifier. The professional component

of the same service can be filed with the NPI of the audiologist, physician, or the non-physician provider (NPP), such as a nurse practitioner, physician's assistant, or certified nurse midwife if they completed the interpretation and report of this service. The reimbursement of these two codes added together is the same as if it were billed globally, meaning that the audiologist, physician, or NPP performed both the test and did the interpretation and report (TC + –26 = global).

The following are requirements to bill "incident to":

- "A procedure or service must be furnished by a physician which initiates the course of treatment;
- The service is billed secondary to the medical visit, or 'incident to' that it is furnished in a non-institutional setting to non-institutional patients; and finally, of
- A type commonly furnished in the office of a physician, furnished under the direct supervision of the physician, furnished by a physician, other practitioner, or auxiliary personnel and only for services that do not have their own benefit category" (CMS, 2013).

Requirements for Audiologists Summary

Currently audiologists have two requirements in the provision of diagnostic services to a Medicare beneficiary: Medical necessity and a physician order. Medical necessity is defined as "reasonable and necessary for the diagnosis or treatment of illness or injury or to improve the functioning of a malformed body member." Medicare requires a physician order due to the physician needing the audiologic information in order to diagnose and treat his or her patient. Change in hearing acuity, balance function, and/or tinnitus should meet medical necessity and the order should indicate the reason for the referral. If specific CPT® codes are ordered, the Medicare policy states that the audiologist can only perform the tests ordered. If another test is necessary for differential diagno-

sis, another order will need to be forthcoming, if it had specific codes requested. If no CPT® codes are specified on the physician order, the audiologist is able to perform the evaluation utilizing the appropriate medically necessary tests to determine the patient's diagnosis and treatment. Medicare will not deny audiologic evaluations if the only diagnosis is sensorineural hearing loss; they will deny the evaluation if the outcome is already known to the physician or the test was ordered for the specific purpose to modify or fit a hearing aid (CMS, 2014). All audiologic procedures and case histories must clearly be documented in the chart as well as signed and dated.

Medicare Enrollment

Audiologists must be enrolled in traditional Medicare Part B. It is advantageous to enroll via the on-line Provider Enrollment Chain, Ownership System (PECOS) at https://pecos.cms.hhs.gov/pecos/login.do as you are able to track the application's status as well as be automatically enrolled in the Medicare Physician Compare website, a consumer-based website designed to provide enrollment information to Medicare beneficiaries who may be in the provider selection process. If a practice chooses to file the Medicare enrollment hard copy form, the 855I, this can also be done with the accompanying 855R form, to reassign the benefits to the employer and should be done whether the audiologist is an employee or contractor. Audiologists can also be part of a group if the group enrolled via the 855B form. Some commercial payers and Medicaid require enrollment in Medicare prior to assigning payment for service.

Prior to 2008, when the Centers for Medicare and Medicaid Services issued Transmittal 84, which specified that the services performed by an audiologist be billed with the NPI of that audiologist, many physicians billed audiologic services to Medicare beneficiaries as "incident to." "Incident to" services have requirements which did not include "other diagnostic tests," the category for audiologic tests. Therefore, the mistaken, pervasive practice of physicians filing claims for services performed by their audiologist-employee with the physician's NPI for the tests performed by that employee should not have been done and should have ceased in 2008.

All audiologic services performed must be filed to Medicare as a result of the Social Security Act (Section 1848(g)(4).

Medicare National and Local Coverage Determination Policies (NCDs and LCDs)

Medicare issues National Coverage Determination (NCD) policies which address appropriate testing and billing practices. The Medicare Administrative Contractors (MACs) have the ability to interpret those national policies and offer local coverage determination policies, which may vary among the MACs. These may be in response to Medicare billing trends. In recent years, several MACs have listed specific CPT® codes and ICD-10 codes that are considered medically necessary and ultimately reimbursable when the required conditions are met. It is imperative that you know what those policies are and where they can be located on your MAC's website. Monitor your MAC's website periodically and subscribe to their e-newsletters notifying providers of upcoming changes, which are usually listed under the headings of "audiologic services," "hearing services," and/or "vestibular disorders." In addition, national professional organizations should be updating members via their websites, e-newsletters, and e-mails.

Advanced Beneficiary Notice

The Advanced Beneficiary Notice (ABN), an alerting notice of the patient's financial responsibility, is a component of the Beneficiary Notices Initiative (BNI). The ABN is designed for the patient to understand that not all of their procedures may be a covered service and informs them of their expected out-of-pocket payment. They have the choice of selecting one of three options on how they choose to have their claim filed.

The first option the patient may choose is to bill Medicare, but you may need to append it with a Medicare specific modifier, described later in this section, if it is for a non-covered service. Due to the mandatory claims statute, you must bill all covered procedures to Medicare. The second option is that the patient understands it is a non-covered service and the claim is not to be filed to Medicare. The third option is that the patient declines the service.

For audiology procedures, there is a mandatory and voluntary use of the ABN. The mandatory ABN informs the patient that the service may not be covered, that it will be filed to Medicare, but if it is denied as "Medicare does not pay for everything, even some care that you or your health care provider have good reason to think you need" (CMS, 2012), then they are responsible. One of the four Medicare specific modifiers (all described below), GA, is used to alert Medicare that the ABN was provided to the patient and they were made aware that the procedure may not be reimbursed. If an ABN is not issued to the patient and the service is denied, the provider is liable and cannot pursue payment from the Medicare beneficiary. A signed and dated ABN must be on file in order to bill the patient if a denial is issued.

The voluntary ABN, which is not required to be offered to the patient but can be, educates the patient about their responsibility for services that are never covered such as hearing aids, cerumen management when performed by an audiologist, and/or any auditory rehabilitative service. While the ABN is not required to be issued for non-covered services, it may be helpful for the patient to understand their fiscal responsibility and the non-coverage of their services.

For example, if the patient's visit is due to an annual routine audiologic evaluation to monitor their hearing acuity, this service is statutorily excluded and a voluntary ABN could be offered to the patient before any services are provided; it notifies them that Medicare will not pay for that particular service. A voluntary ABN could be given to the patient if the visit was due to anything related to hearing aids or rehabilitation, or another service that is statutorily excluded. Medicare should not be billed for any of these non-covered services;

therefore, the patient is financially responsible. But if the patient has a secondary payer which requires a denial from Medicare, you can file the claim to Medicare to obtain the denial with the GY and/or GX modifiers (see Medicare modifiers listed in this chapter). If the patient directs you to bill Medicare for something never covered, again, you may use the GY modifier and not be in violation. Check with your MAC for guidance on the use of the GY and GX modifiers for this scenario.

In wanting to protect your patients and your practice, it is ill advised to have every patient complete an ABN. This is considered to be blanket utilization, is not a recommended policy, and may eventually result in an audit.

You will need to contact your Medicare carrier as local policies differ and therefore contractors may differ in their guidance. The ABN forms and directions can be located on the CMS website (https://www.cms.gov/BNI/02_ABN.asp#TopOfPage).

Medicare Modifiers

Depending on the intent of the claim, there are four Medicare modifiers that you may be required to use: GA, GY, GX, and GZ. Once the Medicare beneficiary chooses one of three options on the ABN, directing how they want their claim to be filed (or not) to Medicare, the provider may then append the modifier(s) to the claim, if necessary.

The Medicare modifiers are described below and include examples of when their use is indicated with audiology procedures.

- GA: "Waiver of Liability Statement issued as Required by Payer Policy," is utilized when a required/mandatory ABN is given to the patient when the audiologist is not certain if the procedures will be covered as they may not be deemed by Medicare to be medically necessary or reasonable. Due to the patient's signature on the ABN attesting they understand their responsibility if a denial is issued, the patient can then be billed for these procedures. Without an ABN and signature, the patient cannot be

billed and the practice will have to write off the claim amount.
- GY: "Item or service statutorily excluded or does not meet the definition of any Medicare benefit," is utilized when the procedure is statutorily excluded and does not meet the definition of a Medicare benefit, such as hearing aids. Many commercial payers require a denial from Medicare in order for the patient to access their hearing aid benefit provided by that secondary payer. In box 19 of the CMS 1500 claim form, you may indicate that this denial by Medicare is necessary in order for the secondary to pay for hearing aids. In combination with the GY modifier, this will prompt an automatic denial. The GY modifier can be appended with another Medicare modifier, the GX modifier, for the same purpose.
- GX modifier: "Notice of Liability Issued, Voluntary Under Payer Policy," indicates a non-required/voluntary ABN, and would be issued for non-covered services such as routine audiologic evaluations that are not based on medical necessity, hearing aids, tinnitus treatment or aural rehabilitation. Patients may be given the voluntary ABN, attesting their understanding of their fiscal responsibility by way of their signature, in case they contest the claim at a later date.
- GZ modifier: "Item or Service Expected To Be Denied As Not Reasonable and Necessary," is utilized when an ABN is not on file, often occurring in an emergent situation. When claims are submitted with this modifier, billing the patient for those services is disallowed and they must be written off. This is the least common Medicare modifier utilized by audiologists.

Physician Quality Reporting System (PQRS) and Merit-Based Incentive Payment System (MIPS)

CMS is transitioning from fee for service (paying for each individual test and encounter) to payment based on outcome measures and other payment paradigms. These methodologies base payment on clinical excellence and care coordination while encouraging fiscal efficiencies.

The Physician Quality Reporting System (PQRS) was designed to be a step in this process. For audiologists it began in 2008 and for all providers, it sunsetted at the end of 2016. Originally instituted as a voluntary program created to improve the quality of care to Medicare beneficiaries while offering an incentive bonus for correct reporting, providers saw the reduction in that bonus over the last few years until the bonus ended in 2014 and a disincentive for not reporting continued to increase. For example, if an audiologist did not report on 50% of Medicare eligible beneficiaries for the measures that had the CPT and ICD-10 code combinations performed, a 2% disincentive was applied to all audiology Medicare reimbursements two years later. There have been a few audiology specific measures over time, some of which were cross-cutting measures on which other professionals may also have reported and included documenting medications, discussing tobacco use, performing depression screenings when performing the tinnitus test (92625), and likely there will more in future methodologies.

At the time of press, the MIPS was in place for physicians but audiologists are not an eligible provider until at least 2019.

Medicare Physician Fee Schedule (MPFS)

Each year, on or around November 1, CMS releases its final rule, detailing payment policy and reimbursement rates for the next year. Each practice should go to the MAC website to obtain those payments to be at the ready for the rates that are supposed to change on January 1 of the following calendar year. This will also position a practice in reviewing these rates in case there are adjustments that need to be made clinically or fiscally.

Claims

Claims are to be made on the CMS 1500 form if filing hard copy. Many audiologists use office man-

agement systems (OMS) which have the capability to do this electronically. This is beneficial to the health of a practice as the claims are submitted in real time, errors are often caught prior to submission, and reimbursement occurs within a few weeks versus the longer time when a hard copy claim is filed.

Medicaid

One cannot mention the CMS without also noting Medicaid programs, which are administered by the state in which the practice resides. If your office is a Medicaid provider, familiarize yourself with the fee schedule, covered services, and applicable otolaryngology and audiology policies, especially for hearing aids. Many states no longer reimburse for hearing aids or for hearing aid evaluations for adults. Due to the Early and Periodic Screening, Diagnostic and Treatment (EPSDT) program responsible for child health, services including hearing aids that meet medical necessity, such as for those who are at risk for hearing loss, are a required covered service for Medicaid beneficiaries from birth to age 21.

Audiologic Technicians/Ototechnicians

Otolaryngology offices may employ audiologic technicians or ototechnicians. In terms of Medicare regulations and audiologic testing as noted above, technicians can only perform the tests that have a technical component (vestibular codes 92537-92546, 92548; comprehensive auditory evoked potentials, diagnostic, 92585, otoacoustic emissions 92587 [limited] and 92588 [comprehensive]). In the initial Medicare transmittal (84) clarifying how to bill for the service of an audiologist, tympanometry was noted as a test that could be performed by a technician, but subsequent transmittals and the Medlearn document 6647, the revision to audiology policies, has not mentioned it again. It is in the best interest of an otolaryngology/audiology or private practice office to clarify this policy as well as the use of the otogram, with your Medicare contractor. A list of Medicare contractors can be located here: http://www.cms.gov/Medicare /Provider-Enrollment-and-Certification/Medicare ProviderSupEnroll/Downloads/contact_list.pdf

Conclusion

This chapter has attempted to offer detailed guidance on billing diagnostic services to Medicare, the most stringent of payers. There are many nuances that are not experienced by other health care providers but are specific to audiologists. It is the hope that this chapter enlightens the staff and the owners of an audiology practice, whether it be a private practice or one housed in an otolaryngology practice, in creating successful and compliant patient services.

References

Centers for Medicare and Medicaid Services. (2013). *Advanced Beneficiary Notice.* Retrieved February 2, 2013, from http:// www.cms.gov/Medicare/Medicare-General-Information /BNI/ABN.html.

Centers for Medicare and Medicaid Services. (2001). *Program Memorandum AB-02-080, Audiologists—Payment for Services Furnished.* Retrieved August 11, 2015, from https:// www.cms.gov/Regulations-and-Guidance/Guidance /Transmittals/downloads/AB02080.pdf.

Centers for Medicare and Medicaid Services. (2008). *Transmittal 84.* Retrieved March 2, 2015, from https://www .cms.gov/transmittals/downloads/R84BP.pdf.

Centers for Medicare and Medicaid Services (April 2013). MLN Matters Number SE 0441. Retrieved August 17, 2015, from https://www.cms.gov/Outreach-and-Education /Medicare-Learning-Network-MLN/MLNMattersArticles /downloads/se0441.pdf.

Centers for Medicare and Medicaid Services (January 2013). MLN Matters Number SE 0908. Retrieved August 17, 2015, from http://www.cms.gov/Outreach-and-Education /Medicare-Learning-Network-MLN/MLNMattersArticles /downloads/SE0908.pdf.

Centers for Medicare and Medicaid Services (January 2013). MLN Matters Number SE 1305. Retrieved March 17, 2016, from https://www.cms.gov/Outreach-and-Education /Medicare-Learning-Network-MLN/MLNMattersArticles /Downloads/se1305.pdf.

Centers for Medicare and Medicaid Services. (2010). *Revisions and re-issuance of Audiology policies-JA6447.* Retrieved August 13, 2015, from http://www.cms.gov/Outreach-and -Education/Medicare-Learning-Network-MLN/MLN MattersArticles/downloads/MM6447.pdf.

Centers for Medicare and Medicaid Services. (2014). *Medicare Benefit Policy Manual, Chapter 15.* Retrieved March 15, 2016, from https://www.cms.gov/Regulations-and-Guidance /Guidance/Manuals/downloads/bp102c15.pdf.

Centers for Medicare and Medicaid Services. (2011). MLN Matters Number: SE0908. Retrieved November 3, 2015, from http://www.cms.gov/MLNMattersArticles/down loads/SE0908.pdf.

Social Security Act. (2003). *Payment for Physician's Services.* Sec. 1848. [42 U.S.C. 1395w–4]. Retrieved July 6, 2015, from http://www.ssa.gov/OP_Home/ssact/title18/1848.htm.

United States Federal Register. (2004). *NPI Final Rule.* Retrieved January 3, 2015, from https://www.cms.gov /Regulations-and-Guidance/Administrative-Simplification /NationalProvIdentStand/Downloads/NPIfinalrule.pdf.

CHAPTER 3

Federal Regulations Applicable to Audiology

Douglas A. Lewis

Introduction

The greatest sources of power for those within any profession are information and knowledge, and the field of clinical audiology is no different. The knowledge acquired from the collection, formulation, and dissemination of relevant information is analogous to the essential building blocks of life often referred to in biological terms as DNA. Just as there are both universal and ascertained laws impacting the natural sciences, there are similar societal and institutional building blocks impacting entire fields of study and practice. These recognized societal "Rules of Law" are essential and sometimes considered necessary evils that often determine how on a macro-level societies and on a more micro-level fields of study and practice are operated and maintained. The Rules of Law are no less important in the arena we define as clinical audiology and are used to establish expected standards of practice and care and thereby formulate and establish formal benchmarks used by a wide range of stakeholders to measure pertinent levels of success or failure in managing our very diverse number of stakeholders while acting in an orderly manner.

The goal of this chapter is to assist audiologists and other relevant stakeholders of care to increase recognition and improve knowledge of the impact of various legal principles, foundations, and parameters for those operating within the hearing healthcare arena. The intent of this chapter is not to represent a legal treatise nor to infer every situation or consideration has a "one size fits all" answer but instead utilizes a broad brush approach when dealing with potential interactions and in some cases collisions between the foundations of our legal system and those influencing hearing healthcare. None of the noted legal context or notations should in any way be construed as legal advice, but instead should be considered as an elucidation of relevant general legal knowledge any individual functioning within the hearing healthcare environment should, with minimal understanding and review, grasp and maintain at minimum a basic working competency in their everyday professional interactions.

Overview

The law has become ingrained as an essential fabric within virtually every part of our lives with the almost endless myriad of media outlets playing their role in communicating, and in some cases "spinning," the impact that legal considerations have on every action and activity in which we participate. Virtually on a daily basis, we're inundated with a multitude of self-proclaimed experts willing to directly or indirectly comment and advise the public on the impact or intent of various laws that could or should influence our decision-making processes or actions. Because of the media hype various legal issues may receive, it would be

33

easy to believe that creating new laws or changing established legal precedents would be a very easy task ("just do it!"—right?). Unfortunately, this belief is a gross oversimplification of an established process and foundation that in some cases has taken hundreds of years (e.g., United States) or even thousands of years (e.g., Europe, Asia) to become established. Over time, most societies have created a very intricate process in the formation and implementation of their legal processes and often refer to or include specific document references which then become the source or foundation for a society's legal and regulatory oversight. The following principles and concepts represent examples of how societies go about establishing the foundation of their respective legal systems.

Established Legal System Structure in the United States

The very essence of democratic governments involves the creation of documents or charters that guide the oversight of their country's affairs. Most democracies (including the United States) rely on an established document such as the Constitution to serve as a roadmap in defining our legal activities, obligations, and behaviors and serves as a backbone or framework for the creation of and conforming to established laws. All is well when legal actions conform to the spirit and intent as noted in the Constitution. However, if certain activities within our legal system violate our Constitutional parameters, those actions can be and generally are struck down or disallowed due to being "unconstitutional."

These constitutional parameters are often written somewhat broadly and not precisely to permit the ongoing enhancement and development of standards that can address changing issues while encompassing a broad spectrum of issues and actions. However, as our society evolves in its social, ethical, and legal evolution, the ability to adapt in meeting changing ethical and legal implications and challenges is essential. The ability to legally enforce our expected standards for societal behavior comes from the creation of laws to further guide our actions.

Black's Law Dictionary defines laws as "a body of rules of action or conduct prescribed by controlling authority, and have binding legal force . . . it is found in its statutory and constitutional enactments, as interpreted by its courts, and in absence of statute law, in rulings of its courts" (Black, 1990). Laws may be created and enacted in different ways including statutes, case law, and executive order. Statutes are laws created by legislative bodies such as the United States Congress (Senate and House of Representatives) as well as at the state level (Senate and House of Representatives) and local representative bodies (e.g., City Councils). Case-made laws are created through adjudication of court cases and the rendering of case decisions within our court systems at the federal, state, and local levels (Figure 3–1). In far fewer cases, the President of the country may create law through the rendering of an Executive Order. Both statutory and case law may be created at the federal, state, and local levels. However, one of the implicit principles mandated by the federal Constitution of different countries is that federal law will always "trump" state law or local law (ordinances) when there are conflicts arising between them resulting in a challenge. Statutory law has also been used to create various agencies to oversee certain functions that may have important societal interests. These agencies may be created to address issues at the federal, state, and local levels with the federal agency rulings again prevailing when conflict arises between "like" agencies at lower levels. The only exceptions to the supremacy characteristic of federal laws trumping lower level statutory, case-made law, or in the rulings of lower like agencies is when the lower level ruling results in a more strict interpretation of the established standards. A more strict interpretation may be necessary to protect our further interests or considerations possessing more importance to a smaller sub-segment of the population by way of certain demographic, geographical, social, or more local considerations. If the lower level ruling "furthers" the interest of the local community and takes a more stringent stance in protecting those interests, the federal Constitution permits the localities to establish these stricter standards. However, under the Supremacy Clause of the United States Constitution, a locality can never weaken

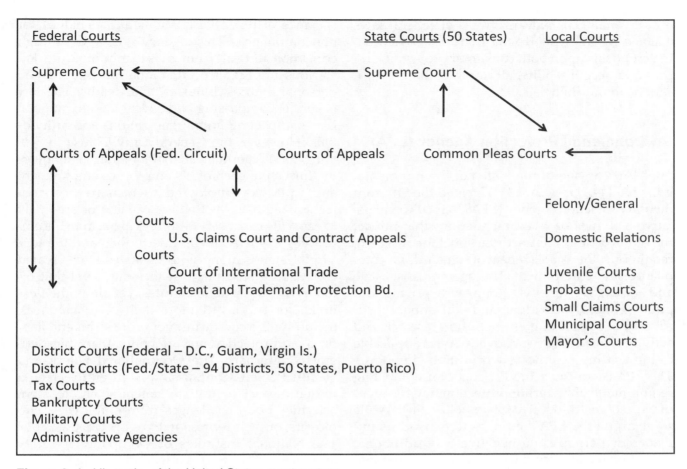

Figure 3–1. Hierarchy of the United States court system.

an established federal standard in an attempt to further its own interests, create some type of local advantage, reduce enforcement capabilities, or create an unhealthy, unsafe, or suboptimal condition that might impact any and all individuals residing, visiting, or performing business or commerce within that locality.

The next level of hierarchy that will influence enforcement of certain legal and regulatory parameters involves actions taken by government-based for-profit or not-for-profit agencies. These agencies may be created to address issues at the federal, state, or local levels with the federal government based agencies again ruling when conflicts arise between "like" agencies at lower levels. Agencies create regulations that are not laws nor have the force of law, but instead are rules created to assist in the governing of their functions. The propagation of these rules and regulations

usually result in the creation of policies and procedures essential for agencies to follow in ensuring actions thereafter are uniform, unbiased, and non-discriminatory in their focus.

Relevant Laws Potentially Impacting Audiologists

Most laws are created with a "broad brush" scope while also delineating the formal oversight authority and/or through court system legal activities that assist in determining compliance or noncompliance. Government and/or non-governmental agencies may be established to ensure laws protecting the public interest are enforced with proper sanctioning authority and activity to address noncompliance. The ensuing sections briefly highlight only a small but relevant group of federal laws enacted by the United States with the overarching emphasis upon both consumer protection and provider accountability, all of which have implications for audiologists.

Environmental Protection Agency (EPA)

The 1970 passage of the National Environmental Policy Act (42 U.S.C.A. 4321) created the Environmental Protection Agency (EPA) to focus on legislative activities or recommendations that impact the environment. EPA activities include research, monitoring, the establishment of standards for compliance, and enforcement. This agency assists state and local governments, along with private and public groups, individual, and educational institutions, in supporting antipollution research and activities, including the relevant issues applicable to the hearing healthcare world involving noise. The EPA established the Product Noise Labeling requirements for hearing protection devices manufactured in the United States (40 CFR). While some argue the EPA continues to expand its bureaucracy perhaps in a negative way, additional educational activities into active noise abatement efforts through education, training, and mandatory warning labels have been established by the EPA's Office of Noise Abatement and Control under the EPA because of the expanding body of evidence of the hazards of high level noise exposure on the human body. Although this particular office does not have enforcement capabilities, it has spawned numerous state efforts into creating and in many cases enforcing local noise regulations.

Occupational Safety and Health Act of 1970 (OSHA)

This federal act created the Occupational Safety and Health Administration (OSHA) with the overarching goal to ensure compliance with written occupational safety and health standards and regulations while ensuring proper investigations and inspections are conducted to affirm organizational and individual compliance with established safety and health regulations, including the

issuance of potential citations and penalties for noncompliance. This agency's charge through education and enforcement is to minimize the deleterious impact of occupational and job-related personal injuries, illnesses, and deaths. The law is very encompassing and covers a wide range of issues impacting both organizations and individuals. However, the General Duty Clause in Section 5(a)(1) is germane in that it requires employers to "furnish to each of his employees employment and a place of employment which are free from recognized hazards that are causing or are likely to cause death or serious physical harm to his employees" (OSHA, 1970). Puerto Rico and the U.S. Virgin Islands along with 24 states have created OSHA-approved plans at the state level that often mirror the federal statutes, yet allow the flexibility for entities to adopt their own standards, including the codification of more stringent standards in protection and sanctions than their federal counterpart. The Occupational Safety and Health Review Commission is an entity created under the act to initiate potential enforcement activities upon challenges from employees, employers, or their representatives (29 U.S.C.A. 661). The National Institutes of Occupational Safety and Health (NIOSH) is a federal U.S. agency created through OSHA that is also an entity within the Centers for Disease Control (CDC) within the U.S. Department of Health and Human Services (DHHS). NIOSH's focus is neither regulatory nor in issuing safety and health standards, but instead to conduct research while developing safety and health regulations focusing on the prevention of work-related illnesses and injury (including those potentially due to hearing and hearing loss considerations). They routinely publish and update numerous bulletins and alerts while managing supporting databases often used in facilitating these and other research activities.

Noise Control Act of 1972

The Noise Control Act was implemented shortly after OSHA's promulgation and delineates the ability for political sub-entities such as cities and states to authorize and implement noise regulation activities at the community level. Over 400-plus cities and other political subdivisions have created and are enforcing noise abatement ordinances where non-compliance can lead to the issuance of citations and other civil sanctions. Noise control goes well beyond simple motor vehicles and can include those emissions from other sound generators such as concerts, community activities, power tools, other operating systems such as heating ventilation or air conditioning systems (HVAC), and many more. States such as California continue to lead the way with many communities now restricting the noise emissions of such routine activities such as gas-powered leaf blowers through the enactment of local ordinances which are further protected under federal statute. The establishment of local restrictions will increase exponentially as the increased recognition of the associated dangers and damage resulting from intense or prolonged noise exposure is documented. OSHA parameters stipulate the requirement of ear protection for prolonged "occupational" exposure beyond 85 dBA for 8 hours of exposure with a 50% decrease in time weighted average (TWA) exposure for every additional 1/2 hour of additional exposure. While the Noise Control Act does not at this time stipulate specific and formal intensity standards regarding noise abatement, many communities are utilizing standards where a maximum sustained intensity level of 60 to 65 dB is referenced with noise levels exceeding these standards being potentially sanctioned under law. Given most smart-phones now have applications ("Apps") that can measure sound levels utilizing a dBA scale, it is not unreasonable to believe the future implications and amendments to this act will continue to proliferate and lead to further enforcement of these laws and others spawning from it.

Health Considerations of Noise Exposure

Our ongoing exposure to many types, levels, and intensity of noise within our environment continue to escalate with our interactions with technology in both occupational and recreational activities. The physical, psychological, emotional, and behavioral effects relating to exposure to adverse levels of noise, especially those occurring at sudden and unexpected levels, are substantial and in many clinical opinions frightening. We are continually exposed to increasingly adverse types and levels of noise from a variety of both unwanted and desired sources including industrial and occupational noise, agricultural endeavors, transportation including air, rail, and motor vehicle traffic, music and entertainment activities, social activities in the community (e.g., restaurants, nightclubs, discos), and our general environment. However, the frequency of use and exposure to a number of desired sources such as concerts, music, personalized systems including MP3 players, and cellular phones continues to increase exponentially as do the numbers of individuals seeking greater and more enhanced access to these items and venues. A value system often perpetuated within our society involves the inference that bigger or more is always better. This attitude is also implied within our acoustic environment and exposure to mean that "louder is better." However, ongoing research in the medical and health science arena is revealing the exact opposite findings in that louder and longer exposures to sound (even wanted or desired sound) can be very risky to one's health as well as potentially to one's pocketbook. This research also routinely reveals direct correlations with the high intensity of various types of noise exposure to health problems including but not exclusive of the following:

- Hearing loss and interruptions with speech communication capabilities
- Tinnitus
- Hypertension (high blood pressure and its effects)
- Vasoconstriction (reduced blood flow)
- Cardiovascular impacts including heart attacks, cardiac arrhythmias, and ischemic heart disease
- Changes in the immune system and birth defects
- Headache
- Fatigue
- Sleep disorders, resting issues, increased body movements in sleep
- Stomach ulcers
- Vertigo and dizziness
- Learning disabilities
- Generalized pain

- Psychological and behavioral stress including increased aggression, depression, and social/antisocial behaviors
- Post-work irritability
- Diminished physical and cognitive performance

There is mounting evidence within the legal literature regarding legal actions commenced by plaintiffs as the result of claimed damage to the audio vestibular system from adverse exposure to noise. Although many claims involve the perceived symptoms as a means to support other claims, there is a growing number of legal claims filed where audio vestibular damage incurred from environmental noise is the primary request for legal relief. The effects of intractable tinnitus and dizziness/vertigo are often so pervasive, devastating, and increasing at an exponential rate with cases being brought forth highlighting the practice of individuals seeking relief through pharmacological self-medication or overmedication, substance abuse, and even suicide. Many psychological and acoustic studies have confirmed the deleterious impacts high noise levels have on individuals living near airports, factories, and even within the busy inner city. The number of Workers' Compensation cases being filed due to physical and mental conditions emanating from some level of overexposure to extremely loud working environments is increasing with many often claiming emotional distress causing psycho-physiological symptoms previously noted including immunocompromised body systems, cardiovascular issues, and stomach ulcers among others. The ability to achieve and maintain adequate sleep because of excessive noise exposure is a growing problem, especially in the achievement of essential slow wave sleep and rapid eye movement (REM), sleep states necessary for proper physiological and psychological well-being. Although sleep disorders are not currently recognized as a protected condition under the Americans with Disabilities Act (ADA) as an essential life activity or function, one cannot doubt the eventual attempts at obtaining legal protection and hence remedies at law through recognition of inadequate acquisition of sleep and the related associated disorders due to the impact of noise exposure as a result of efforts espoused in societal and public policy initiatives. The presence of adverse and/or excessive noise exposure being the nexus or connection is one being seriously considered in many legal analyses as viable arguments to support these claims. The likely nexus of adverse noise exposure due to the loss of sleep along with many other psychophysiological anomalies cannot be understated or dismissed within the legal arena and will almost ensure future litigation efforts, time and financial expenditures, loss of societal productivity, and a likely degradation of the quality of life for those adversely impacted. All of these components have a direct impact on audiologists and those served by audiologists.

Ongoing research has affirmed the routine presence of the aforementioned health issues within average or normal populations. However, studies of the impacts upon perceived vulnerable populations such as the elderly, the very young, and people already possessing certain physical, emotional, or cognitive disabilities will continue to move forward as data continues to be acquired, mined, and analyzed. Given the compromised state of most of these individuals for a whole host of other reasons, it would be easily inferred that the scope and magnitude of the reduced capabilities to cope with adverse impacts of noise exposure would be compounded many times over and would result in members of those vulnerable populations being at even a greater risk from the harmful effects of such exposure.

The Americans with Disabilities Act of 1990 (ADA)

The ADA built upon prior enacted legislative mandates protecting potential discriminatory practices that include but are not exclusive of Title VII of the 1964 Civil Rights Act, The Age Discrimination in Employment Act of 1967, and the Pregnancy Discrimination Act of 1978. The ADA was specifically created to ensure that "no individual shall be discriminated against on the basis of disability in the full and equal employment of the goods, services, facilities, privileges, advantages, or accommodations of any place or public accommodation" (American Disabilities Act of 1990). Audiologists can directly be impacted by the guidelines and parameters of the ADA in dealing with potential individuals protected under its auspices because of the following considerations:

1. To provide a clear and *comprehensive national mandate* for the elimination of discrimination versus individuals with disabilities;
2. To provide clear, strong, consistent, and *enforceable standards* addressing discrimination versus individual with disabilities;
3. To *ensure the federal government plays a central role in enforcing standards* established in the Act on behalf of individuals with disabilities; and
4. To *involve the sweep of congressional authority,* including the power to enforce the 14th Amendment of the U.S. Constitution both federally and at the state level and to regulate commerce in order to address the major areas of discrimination faced daily by people with disabilities (ADA, 1990).

The ADA is designed to protect against discriminatory practices against individuals possessing disabilities in one or more of the following major life activities:

- Breathing
- Walking
- Learning
- Seeing
- Working
- Caring for oneself
- Hearing

The ADA has several subsections to it, but it does address several important hearing considerations in the following manner:

1. Title I articulates a methodology to ensure that individuals with covered disabilities have the same opportunities for employment as people without disabilities. Employers with 15 or more employees are required to provide reasonable accommodations to the person with a disability to allow them to perform their job. This law does not ensure jobs, but rather prohibits discrimination in employment for people who are qualified to carry out the "essential" functions of a specific job.
2. Title II requires that state and local governmental agencies make their programs accessible to people with disabilities, including transportation programs. Effective communication for deaf and hard-of-hearing people must be ensured and auxiliary aids must be provided. Such aids include, but are not limited to, assistive listening systems, qualified interpreters, captioning, provision of TTYs and amplified telephones, text displays, and transcription of audio programs.
3. Title III requires that public places (operated by private entities) including private business, professional offices, and not-for-profit organizations provide communication access. The list of those affected is extensive and includes the following: hotels, restaurants, movie theaters, stadiums, concert halls, retail stores of all types, transportation terminals, museums, libraries, senior centers, sports facilities, and swimming pools. Required accommodations include the aids listed above in Title II as well as television decoders and visual alerting devices (in hotel rooms). The ADA Accessibility Guidelines, first developed by the Access Board in 1991, provided specific requirements for certain accommodations to be provided in new construction and renovation of existing structures (such as assistive listening technology in theaters and other facilities, visual alerting devices in hotel rooms, TTY, and accessible pay phones in public places).
4. Title IV requires that all telephone companies provide relay services throughout the United States. Such services must be provided on a 24/7 basis. Individuals may not be charged for such services and there are no restrictions on the length or nature of the calls.

ADA mandates compliance with those either receiving federal funds or participating in federal programs. However, the federal ADA is merely a "floor" creating an expected minimal level of compliance. Most states now have their own versions of the ADA that must be no less encompassing but are generally considerably more encompassing regarding public protection and sanction capabilities. Audiologists involved in the area of hearing aid dispensing and assistive-listening devices (ALDs) should maintain a working understanding of several ensuing laws that have since spawned from the parameters of the ADA including the following:

- Hearing Aid Compatibility Act requires that all "essential" telephones manufactured after August 16, 1989 be compatible for use with hearing aids. The definition of compatible was changed and expanded to include a requirement for a volume control. ANSI standards provide a methodology for "essential" telephones requiring the notation of a ratings scale from M1 to M4 that delineates compatibility with hearing aids with M1 being the least immune to radio-frequency interference and M4 being the most immune. The level of interference to immunity is calculated based on a summation of ratings. A summation of the hearing aid to telephone rating of four indicates the telephone is usable whereas a sum of five would indicate that the telephone would be viable for basic normal use. A sum of six or greater would indicate that the telephone would provide excellent performance when used in combination with the hearing aid.
- Individuals with Disabilities Education (IDEA) requires that children with disabilities be provided with a free and appropriate public education that includes special education and related services to meet the "unique" needs of children, including the establishment of ongoing Individualized Education Program (IEP) Plans. Safeguards were built into the act to allow parents to pursue remedies if their local schools do not meet their child's needs. State and local governments are required to provide education for children through grade 12 in the United States and the law applies to public (not private) educational institutions.
- Television Decoder Circuitry Act requires all television sets with screens 13 inches or larger, manufactured or imported into the United States after July 1, 1993, to be capable of displaying closed-captioned television transmissions. All TVs must use specific and uniform display standards addressing the placement, italics, background, use of upper- and lower-

case lettering, and proper manufacturer's labeling.
- Rehabilitation Act of 1973 (with subsequent amendments) requires that programs receiving federal funds can be used by people with disabilities, thus the federal government cannot operate in a discriminatory manner. Any grant, loan, or contract to an entity or program, public or private, requires that entity to follow the regulations of the act.
- Telecommunications Act of 1996 requires television programming including broadcast, cable, and satellite to follow a specific schedule to provide captioning. Although there are specific exemptions (e.g., programming shown between 2 a.m. and 6 a.m. local time, programming in languages other than English and Spanish), all new nonexempt programming must be captioned. This act also requires telecommunications products and services to be accessible to and usable by people with disabilities, if readily achievable to do so. A major focus of concern for hard-of-hearing and deaf people after passage of this act was digital wireless telephone services, which often interfere with hearing technology and are not compatible with text telephones (TTYs).

Potential Legal Ramifications and Consequences of Noise-Induced Hearing Loss

There is an enormous amount of research that reveals many correlations between higher exposures to noise levels through participation in activities and our surrounding environment inflicting many adverse effects on humans through various physical, psychological, and emotional conditions. Numerous legislative initiatives have been proffered to try to address these concerns through not only education but with sanctions for non-compliance with known adverse conditions. Despite these initiatives, adverse consequences resulting in hearing health care issues are on the increase due to exposure to yet louder occupational and recreational environments. The number and magnitude of impairment levels continue to soar due to exposure to damaging noise.

The social, political, and economic challenges confronted by individuals experiencing hearing system deficits has been well researched and documented. While some of these challenges are the result of congenital or inherited traits or conditions, many more are being connected to various noise and noise exposure issues within our environment. Although positive changes are occurring in certain societal values and mores regarding noise reduction, many of these changes continue to lag or are often implemented far too slowly and may often be watered-down in their impact after so-called "legislative efforts." As a result, many individuals who perceive that their rights to protection from adverse conditions due to inactivity in implementing protective measures, the lack of actual measures, or the possible inadequacy or defect in their construction often will choose to resort to legally based efforts to seek remedies for conditions they perceive as being responsible for causing their impediment or deficit. These concerns are legitimate and must be taken seriously by all parties potentially responsible for the safety and well-being of our acoustic environment.

A host of potential legal actions may be considered by the alleged aggrieved party when a perceived hearing injury has occurred. Many of the potential remedies are obvious and often pleaded while other perhaps more novel and exotic are being utilized more to perhaps set a landmark precedent for the "triers of fact" (courts or other adjudicating bodies) to consider in addressing complaints and perhaps crafting remedies. No pleaded remedy should be considered on its face as without merit and can represent legitimate concerns and activities and should be viewed as potential legal actions when an injury or deficit has occurred.

Many current laws and agency actions have been implemented and/or are mandated because of available research indicating problematic occupationally related noise environments. Most organizations are very aware of and conscious in their efforts to ensure available safety options are in place and generally comply with the best of intentions and in good faith. However, established mech-

anisms of actions to address non-compliance regardless of motivation must be available. Most organizations with employees as well as outside contractors and vendors are responsible to participate in safety initiatives. However when non-compliance does occur, the motivation of the non-compliant can have significant implications regarding potential sanctions and remediation activities or requirements. The aggrieved may resort to activities such as "whistle-blowing" when they perceive their voices are not being heard. Whistleblowers generally are alleging misconduct in the workplace through known or perceived illegal or otherwise unacceptable actions or behaviors such as violations of laws, rules, regulations, and/or a direct threat to public interest, such as fraud, health/safety violations, and/or corruption. One of the requirements for whistle-blowing is the need to show their duress either directly or through implication to violate standards or being threatened in some manner should they not conform to the overseer's improper motivations. An example could involve working in an environment where the level of noise exposure knowingly exceeds OSHA standards, but yet are warned and/or are threatened with retaliation for complaining or disclosing. Whistleblowers often have a myriad of motivators for their actions; many are legitimate and even admirable (like doing the right thing), others may be more personally driven in their motivation (like sticking it to 'the man' or for financial compensation). There are certain established legal protections for whistleblowers if the complaint is valid and if it falls under federal protection of the Whistleblower Protection Act, the No Fear Act, or the Military Whistleblower Act among others. Other potential limited protections include the Sarbanes-Oxley Act, Anti-Kickback Statutes, and the False Claims Act, as well as a number of existing state statutes, and any existing company rules or policies. Regardless of their motivation, the whistleblower can endure considerable personal, professional, and financial risks including, but not exclusive of, termination of employment, loss of relationships and affiliations. An important consideration in the hearing health care arena for potential whistleblowing activities is when parameters of hearing conservation programs are not being followed when they simply do not exist. The parameters are many, but could include such actions as a lack of or insufficient program oversight, monitoring, or compliance, lack of available appropriate hearing protective devices, lack of readily available acoustic shielding, or overexposure to adverse sound levels. Whistle-blowing often will result in certain civil remedies including monetary fines, injunctions, or "cease and desist orders." Whistle-blowing or the potential thereof must be considered as a very serious consideration and *never* taken lightly because of the safety and health considerations and the potential resultant hearing impairment issues.

Tort Law

Tort law is an area of law that has both great concern and great opportunities to create real impacts on both providers and consumers within the hearing health care arena. Torts come in all shapes and sizes with some being considered worse than others. Tort claims are civil court claims and generally do not hold any criminal implications or liability. The plaintiff in a tort action must successfully meet and prove the existence of the following four elements for their case to be successful against the interests of a defendant:

- Duty
- Breach
- Causation or nexus (direct connection)
- Damages

The first element involves the requirement that an ascertainable duty to do or not do something actually existed. If there is no duty or requirement to perform an action, then one cannot sustain a claim of tort liability.

The second element involves a breach or violation of an ascertained duty. If one legally possesses an ascertained duty to do or not to do something and willfully does not comply with said duty, then an obvious breach of that duty exists. For example, if one is to perform a certain procedure or action and simply chooses not to do it regardless of their motivation, then there is a breach of that duty. Another means of breaching a duty

is through omission of the performance of some particular task or protocol. Again, motivation for the omission is irrelevant whether it is purely accidental or unintentional because it is nonetheless a breach of that duty. Non-performance of a duty due to ignorance is also not a viable excuse and is a breach if that duty is part of the accepted or expected standard of action or care. Where the motivation regarding the type of breach does play a role is in the differentiation of the concepts of *simple* negligence or *gross* negligence which will be explained shortly.

The third essential element of negligence involves causation or nexus. One claiming the occurrence of a tort must prove that the duty and breach of that duty was directly connected to the claimed injury. Merely acknowledging the presence of an articulated injury as well as a potential breach of an ascertainable duty is still not enough to prove tort liability unless one can show the injury was the actual result of the breached duty and not either incidental or coincidental to the breach. Claimed injuries may be caused by multiple sources, but if one cannot show a definitive connection or causality between the breached duty and the injury, then any direct claims of liability under tort will legally fail.

The fourth element is damages. Damages are claim for relief in an attempt to make the claimant or their injury "whole" or as if the incident never happened. This relief routinely comes in the form of damages. There are a number of damages that may be pled in a tort suit with the compensatory damages to make the claimant whole being the essential ones. Periodically punitive damages may also be claimed to "punish" the offender or their offensive action and usually involves a request for a very high level of monetary compensation. The concepts of simple and gross negligence play a role in this determination. Simple negligence is relatively easy to prove, especially if the ascertained duty and breach of said duty is obvious and an obvious connection of the injury to that breached duty can be proven. Gross negligence comes into play when the action/inaction results in a significant or catastrophic injury and the motivation for the negligence was very inappropriate up to the point of actions being extremely or grossly inadequate, improper, and such a violation of care that it would "shock the conscience" of even a reasonable person.

There are several different categories of torts. The list of intentional torts continues to grow as our laws evolve, especially those where changes in perceived societal ethical values previously deemed not illegal but perceived as so unethical they should be sanctioned. Some of those with potential implications to hearing loss from the committing of intentional torts include the following:

- Battery (unwanted physical touching)
- Assault (placed in immediate apprehension of injury)
- Intentional infliction of emotional distress (intentionally causing some physical or psycho-physiological injury through one's actions)

The following is a very brief list of examples of torts where an audiologist may become involved not only clinically in the identification of possible consequences resulting from a tort action but also perhaps in the requirement to participate in any following legal activities based on their findings or perhaps as an "expert witness" in determining cause and effect:

- The effects of a firecracker thrown at or near someone with an intent to explode near them resulting in hearing loss or other damage (regardless of the motivation);
- Horseplay at an industrial site with machinery such as air compressors and nozzles near the ears (this author litigated a case with similar circumstances to this one);
- Turning the volume of a piece of equipment up loud so it blasts full when turned on thereby scaring the individual and resulting in some claimed injury;
- Smacking someone hard on their ears with an open palm or cupped hands; and so on.

Strict liability is a classification of torts involving liability without fault and because the obvious issues rarely require the need for expert testimony.

These are activities producing liability without fault where one does not have to prove fault, complicity, or negligence. Relevant examples may include the following:

- Ultra-hazardous activities (blasting or other exposure to known high intensity sounds)
- Workers' Compensation (routine work exposure in loud areas such as factories, flight lines, military, etc.)
- Warranties and representations (manufacturer warranties or representations that are not followed by the manufacturer or provider on equipment (i.e., hearing aids, assistive listening devices, ear-level music players)
- Reasonable misinterpretation by the public due to lack of supplied education or information regarding the proper use of equipment or products

Products liability is often a consideration when consumers claim injury from a perceived defect with such problems as improper packaging, instructions for use, component composition, or output generation (i.e., electricity or sound of a product such as amplification devices, portable ear level devices, etc. that malfunction or are improperly made that result in damage to the hearing mechanism). A lack of or missing manufacturer warnings on the devices may also result in claims of liability from a potentially defective product when some injury or damage is shown. A real-world example applicable to the profession could involve the manufacturer of a toy gun whose sound emissions mimic a real gun's output at 125 dB of sound resulting in enormous liability risks to its users and any others around it during operation. Another possible products liability scenario could involve the production of MP3 players with no warning labels regarding the potential range of sound emissions and with no manual or preset limitations to the level of sound/music and delivered through insert or other earphones/earbuds that could easily result in significant damage to the hearing system. The legal sale of fireworks and related noisemakers emitting excessively loud impact sounds also create a real risk both to the consumer and to the seller. This becomes an ongoing risk management issue for product producers in creating a viable product for consumer use that will be desired and utilized, but at the same time safe for use. Internal process review, assessment, and monitoring activities are imperative as is proactive identification and action when issues are discovered. On the other hand, consumers must be willing and desire to utilize the product and understand that all products generally produce a certain level of inherent risk in their use. Non-meritorious or frivolous complaints can result in unnecessary recalls and/or elimination of products that are otherwise reasonably safe if properly used.

Workers' Compensation Programs

Another strict liability consideration potentially resulting from the adverse effects on hearing or related impairments involves claims through administration of Workers' Compensation programs. These programs have been put in place to specifically ensure that workers are protected from injuries determined to have been sustained in the workplace *regardless* of what happened or who might have been at fault. Workers' Compensation programs mandate employers automatically pay into the system whether they may have claims or not. There is no provision requiring the determination of fault to be eligible for injury compensation as long as the injury is shown to have resulted from some activity either directly involved in the workplace or verifiably linked to it. This program serves multiple purposes for both the injured individual and the organization. The injured individual is not required to pay for injuries sustained within the workplace and generally assumes no other liability or responsibility other than returning where possible to their prior state of health with no loss of employment, seniority, or other previously eligible benefits. Simultaneously, the organization is able to pay for costs associated with that worker's injury from a shared risk pool they are mandated to pay into and permits a sharing of said risk by all other organizations paying into it. This reduces the financial burden on the organization

in question and allows funding from a greater pool of contributions while spreading risk. There are additional benefits in that programs offering safe work environments can obtain reduced payments into the Workers' Compensation program pool by maintaining low claims and minimal dispersements. The incentive is significant and can result in a substantial financial saving for organizations. Additionally, other insurance premiums organizations that involve safety parameters may be positively impacted by their lower Workers' Compensation "Experience Ratings."

One potential downside for injured workers involves the attempt to bring legal claims against the organization. If they are injured and are participating in the Workers' Compensation program, they're being compensated for their injury with a goal of making them "whole" as if no injury had occurred. Although participation does not preclude an employee from filing other legal claims against the employer, the fact that they are already benefiting from participation in the Workers' Compensation program can be introduced into the proceedings. Many courts are routinely hesitant to further claims they determine will result in a potential windfall for the person filing them who is already fully participating and receiving benefits through programs such as the Workers' Compensation program.

Unintentional torts are perhaps the most common yet often the most feared because they often simply occur without obvious intent to injure or willful non-compliance. Perhaps the one most common yet problematic for audiologists to be concerned with involves the tort of negligence. Negligence results from liability due to a perceived breach of a defined duty to act within a certain set of standards, parameters, or scope of activity. The concepts of simple and gross negligence play a role in this determination. Simple negligence is not difficult to prove, especially if the duty is ascertainable with an obvious breach and an obvious connection of the injury to that breached duty. Gross negligence comes into play when the action/inaction has resulted in significant injury and the motivation for the negligence was very inappropriate such that the actions were extremely or grossly inadequate, improper, and were such a violation of care that it would "shock the conscience" of even a reasonable person.

Relevant examples of potential negligence actions may include the following:

- Negligent infliction of emotional distress (emotional distress resulting from negligent actions by a professional or non-professional) where a verifiable injury has occurred, such as worsening of a hearing loss, damage to the hearing or balance anatomy causing a verifiable physical injury, and so on.
- Professional malpractice (improper or willful negligence from a health care professional through deviation of an accepted standard of care resulting in damage or the furthering of damage to the audio vestibular mechanism). This could include prescribing ear level devices resulting in over-amplification, a failure or omission to properly inform a patient regarding the use of devices, ear protection, battery care, improper earmold impression procedures, and so on.

General non-professional negligence is also classified through the determination of actions that comprise either simple or gross negligence. Any action taken outside the professional realm that deviates from those expected of a reasonable person that results in some ascertainable injury or damage is negligence. Horseplay resulting in injury to the ears is sadly all too common. The failure to supply proper ear protection resulting in damage is an example of negligence. However, if an intent to not properly supply said protection was due to being reckless, willful, wanton, or even a financial basis (didn't want to spend the money) and the lack of supplying it resulted in ascertainable damage to one's hearing mechanism, a claim of gross negligence (reckless disregard) would be a potential and valid claim. If gross negligence is proven in court, the civil monetary penalties can be enormous!

Depending on the scope and severity of the alleged tort, the potential to make inferences and connect tort actions to those much greater could

lead one into criminal court if not careful. The difference between them is that a civil wrong is an action brought by one against another whereas a criminal complaint is one brought by a governmental actor or subdivision such as the state or federal government against a private person as a result of a perceived "injury" against the public or public interest. Both have dramatically different motivations and anticipated remedies. Civil claims often involve the request for a legal remedy such as financial compensation or an injunction (cease and desist order), a request for contract reformation, or other civil processes. Criminal claims may involve monetary reimbursement, but are usually also tied to some type of incarceration or significant penalty above and beyond a simple request for financial or injunctive expectations.

Another curious legal consideration that hearing and noise issues could potentially trigger liability involves the violation of a property and contract law principle known as Quiet Enjoyment. This is a matter that organizations, property owners, and even tenants should consider as a possible issue when dealing with noise complaints regarding their activities when in the presence of others in these facilities. The increasing impact and focus on noise pollution and complaints and other environmental issues can realistically lead to complaints regarding one's inability under a contract right to be able to enjoy their "quiet and solitude" in their dwelling or occupancy of their land and represents a potential legal risk that could be quantified and may result in more court-requested claims for relief. Claims may not only include individual parties seeking redress from other individuals, but perhaps individuals against organizations and/or political subdivisions and vice versa. Many of the noise abatement laws and statutes have been promulgated to meet these new and growing potential issues impacting hearing health care.

Anti-Kickback Statute

The Federal Anti-Kickback Statute [42 U.S.C. s 1320-7b (b)] and its related corollary laws adapted by the respective states "prohibit anyone from knowingly and willfully soliciting and receiving any remuneration (payment including any kickback, bribe, or rebate) directly or indirectly, overtly or covertly, in cash or in kind in return for referring an individual or another person or entity for a service that may be paid by any federally funded health care program regardless of the intent for the referral" (CMS, 1991). This implicit benefit can include purchases, leases, orders, or arranging for or recommending purchases thereof; facility usage, or items for which payment may be made in whole or in part under a federal health care program in return for improper remuneration where there is an implication of benefit for the referrer regardless of the tangibility of said benefit or the intent of the referral. Civil and criminal monetary penalties may be assigned with civil penalties up to $50,000 for each violation with the potential for treble damages. Criminal monetary penalties of up to $25,000 and up to five years of incarceration can also be levied against the offenders. There are many activities that could impute potential liability for audiologists including but not exclusive of the following:

- Directly compensating another practitioner (i.e., physicians, nurse practitioners) based on the number of referrals sent which ultimately result in revenue billed and collected from a governmental entity or one doing business with the government.
- Splitting reimbursements with referral sources based on the number or quality of said referrals.
- Entering into agreements to lease or rent space from another based on referral numbers sent to you or perhaps for preferential pricing resulting in a "sweetheart deal" that is well below fair market value (FMV) or perhaps even free.

Any arrangement where there is compensation that is not fixed based on an accepted parameter in occupying space such as a fixed dollar per time frame or based on size (i.e., square footage) where the compensation is variable and numbers driven could potentially invoke liability under either the Federal Anti-Kickback Statute or a potential state correlative version of the law (CMS, 2012).

Federal False Claims Act

The Federal False Claims Act (FCA; 31 U.S.C. sections 3729-3733) was originally created in 1863 during the Civil War to prosecute individuals billing for and in some cases stealing from and reselling stolen Union Army property back to the federal government for personal gain at the expense of the government. As in the above-referenced corollary Anti-Kickback Statute, the FCA also has related state versions that may create additional potential liabilities for offenders beyond and/or in addition to the basic federal considerations. The spirit and intent live on today as the law has evolved into prosecuting improper and/or frivolous claims for services with the intent of obtaining remuneration from the federal government (i.e., Medicare, Medicaid, or other third-party payers with a government contract) for services either performed inadequately, improperly, or not at all. Claims may be considered false for a variety of reasons including but not exclusive of if the service is not actually rendered to the patient, is provided but already covered under another claim, is miscoded, or is not supported by the medical record. The two primary areas of interest that may evoke scrutiny under this law involve those falling under the auspices of "Worthless Service" and the other involving "Implicit Certification" of services performed but in a defective or improper matter and thereby receiving remuneration for said services. This law encourages the volunteering of information against the potential offender in assisting the prevention of fraud against the government and provides strong incentive for the aforementioned "whistle-blowers" to report fraud. These whistle-blower suits are known as "qui tam" actions and can be quite lucrative to the whistle-blower. If the government proceeds against the accused provider of service on the basis of the information received, the whistle-blower will receive 15% of any service reimbursement plus penalties received by the government from the offending service provider. Should the government not initially pursue the case, but instead the whistle-blower retains private counsel who moves the claim forward and ultimately wins the judgment, then the whistle-blower and his legal representatives will receive up to 30% of the damages assessed by the government.

Hence, the incentives for qui tam actions moving forward on accusations of false claims filings by the government are significant.

Examples of potential false claims may include activities involving:

- Overbilling
- Billing for services not rendered
- Unbundling one item into several claims or unbundling a bundled code that is otherwise prohibited under law
- Upcoding services for higher reimbursement
- Providing inferior products
- Paying kickbacks for referrals (often also prosecuted under the Anti-Kickback Statute)
- Falsifying claims and medical records to certify patients for benefits they otherwise could not receive or would be ineligible to receive
- Billing for ghost patients or phantom services
- Duplicate submissions of the same service or claim
- Payments for excluded or medically unnecessary services
- Patterns of furnishing and billing for excessive or non-covered services
- Billing for false diagnosis of audio vestibular disorders that do not exist or are not clinically verifiable

Two particular subcategories of potential liability audiologists should be concerned with involve rendering care and receiving compensation for services deemed to be "Worthless Service" or due to "Implicit Certification." "Worthless service" involves performing testing services or procedures that do not appear to render any additional benefit in either the diagnosis or treatment of an audio vestibular condition but are nonetheless billed for and reimbursed. Another potential worthless service would involve performing activities that actually contribute to the worsening of a condition (i.e., increasing the severity of a noise-induced hearing loss due to improper amplification) could potentially be inferred as a worthless service. "Implicit Certification" involves the verification through documentation where the audiologist notes a certain result of their testing, bills, and receives reimbursement, but the test results are incorrect due to improper technique or equipment use. One real concern with this scenario involves the use of diagnostic equipment that is perhaps not in proper working order due to being dysfunctional in some way or perhaps having not been nor ever been professionally maintained and/or calibrated. The audiologist could be implicated for liability for a false claim if they use faulty equipment to obtain results which may be erroneous due to the faulty equipment yet obtain reimbursement for services rendered with said equipment.

The FCA carries some very strict sanctions and penalties for non-compliance. Civil monetary penalties may range from $5,000 to $11,000 per false claim which can potentially be *tripled* per claim depending on the severity plus the costs of prosecution. Additionally, criminal penalties of up to five years and prison and up to $10,000 in fines, or both, can exist.

Enforcement under the FCA may also be invoked in conjunction with Section 6402 of the Patient Protection and Affordable Care Act (PPACA) of 2010 which requires providers (including audiologists) to report and return federal overpayment of services to their relevant Medicare contractor within 60 days of identifying the overpayment. Furthermore, intent is *not required* to evoke scrutiny under the FCA and liability can be imputed even from an honest mistake! Practitioners are strongly encouraged to adopt strict compliance and risk assessment programs that focus on ensuring thorough and timely documentation, the performance of internal audits and reviews of billed services, the utilization of third-party external audits, the encouragement of employee self-reporting of discovered mistakes or concerns without fear of reprisal, and the appointment of a designated compliance officer or person responsible in oversight of these activities.

Stark Law

The Stark Physician Self-Referral Laws (42 CFR 411.351-357) are violated when physicians refer federally funded patients (e.g., Medicare and Medicaid) to entities where they or other close family members have a financial relationship outside a recognized safe harbor. These entities include financial ownership, investment, or compensation relationships with an entity providing "designated health services," which are prohibited from billing for the provision of services provided based on a prohibited referral. While there are many "designated service" prohibitions including various imaging, radiation, laboratory, DME, and a variety of outpatient services, audiology is not one of those specific services at the time of this publication. One of the primary concerns involves the level of physician involvement if the physician is a close family member to the audiologist and essentially "automatically" refers their patients to said audiologist because of the family connection *without* either putting the patient on notice of said relationship or affording the opportunity for patients to choose from a list of providers that can include the audiologist regardless of the familial connection. While the audiologist would not likely have any direct liability under Stark Laws, if the inference involves physician ownership of the practice, potential liability may not fall under a Safe Harbor Exception protection. One other possible imputed liability involves the issue of *Fair Market Value*. This can be connoted if there is a relationship where the physician either rents or leases space to the audiologist that is well below established market value (or the relationship is reversed and the audiologist is the tenant and physician is the lessee). This implies an unfair relationship where the physician and those affiliated parties are mutually benefiting in an improper manner. Additionally, should a relationship exist where there is any "payment for referrals" relationships flowing in either direction through this landlord-tenant relationship, a violation of the aforementioned Anti-Kickback Statutes may also exist simultaneously. Application of this standard results in the violation rising to a level of a strict liability standard where no actual fault is required to prove non-compliance. Potential violations may include civil monetary penalties up to $15,000 per each improperly submitted claim. Additionally, if the providers entered into arrangements known to willingly circumvent referral restriction laws, the penalties could rise to

$100,000 per arrangement plus potential exclusion from participating in federally funded programs including Medicare and Medicaid.

Health Insurance Portability and Accountability Act of 1996 (HIPAA)

The Health Insurance Portability and Accountability Act of 1996 (HIPAA), Public Law 104-191, was enacted on August 21, 1996. Sections 261 through 264 of HIPAA require the Secretary of Health and Human Services (HHS) to publicize standards for the electronic exchange, privacy, and security of health information. Collectively these are known as the Administrative Simplification provisions. It required the secretary of HHS to develop regulations protecting the privacy and security of certain health information. To fulfill this requirement, HHS published what are commonly known as the HIPAA Privacy Rule and Security Rules. The Privacy Rule, or Standards for Privacy of Individually Identifiable Health Information, establishes national standards for the protection of certain health information known as PHI (Protected Health Information). The Security Standards for the Protection of Electronic Protected Health Information (the Security Rule) establish a national set of security standards for protecting certain health information that is held or transferred in electronic form. The Security Rule operationalizes the protections contained in the Privacy Rule by addressing the technical and non-technical safeguards that organizations called "covered entities" must put in place to secure individuals' "electronic protected health information" (e-PHI). Within HHS, the Office for Civil Rights (OCR) has responsibility for enforcing the Privacy and Security Rules with voluntary compliance activities and civil money penalties.

HIPAA Privacy Rule

A major goal of the Privacy Rule is to assure that individuals' health information is properly protected while allowing the flow of health information needed to provide and promote quality health care and to protect the public's health and well-being. The Rule strikes a balance that permits important uses of information, while protecting the privacy of people who seek care. The Rule is designed to be flexible and comprehensive to cover the variety of uses and disclosures that need to be addressed. The Privacy Rule, as well as all the Administrative Simplification rules, applies to health plans, health care clearinghouses, and to any health care provider who transmits health information in electronic form in connection with transactions for which the Secretary of HHS has adopted standards under HIPAA, known as "covered entities." Any audiologist who electronically transmits health information in connection with certain transactions is a covered entity. These transactions include claims, benefit eligibility inquiries, referral authorization requests, or other transactions for which HHS has established standards under the HIPAA Transactions Rule. Using electronic technology, such as email, does not mean a health care provider is a covered entity; the transmission must be in connection with a standard transaction. The Privacy Rule covers an audiologist whether they electronically transmit transactions directly from their own office software or use a billing service or other third party to do so on their behalf.

Business Associate Agreements

An audiologist is considered a business associate if they are other than a member of a covered entity's workforce, who performs certain functions or activities on behalf of, or provides certain services to, a covered entity that involves the use or disclosure of individually identifiable health information. Business associate functions or activities on behalf of a covered entity include claims processing, data analysis, utilization review, and billing. Business associate services to a covered entity are limited to legal, actuarial, accounting, consulting, data aggregation, management, administrative, accreditation, or financial services. However, persons or organizations are not considered business associates if their functions or services do not involve the use or disclosure of protected health information, and where any access to protected health information by such persons would be in-

cidental, if at all. A covered entity can be the business associate of another covered entity. When a covered entity uses a contractor or other non-workforce member to perform "business associate" services or activities, the Rule requires that the covered entity include certain protections for the information in a business associate agreement (in certain circumstances governmental entities may use alternative means to achieve the same protections). In the business associate contract, a covered entity must impose specified written safeguards on the individually identifiable health information used or disclosed by its business associates. Moreover, a covered entity may not contractually authorize its business associate to make any use or disclosure of protected health information that would violate the Rule.

Personal Health Information (PHI)

The Privacy Rule protects all "individually identifiable health information" held or transmitted by a covered entity or its business associate, in any form or media, whether electronic, paper, or oral. The Privacy Rule calls this information "protected health information (PHI)." "Individually identifiable health information" is information, including demographic data, that relates to:

- The individual's past, present, or future physical or mental health or condition,
- The provision of health care to the individual, or
- The past, present, or future payment for the provision of health care to the individual, and that identifies the individual or for which there is a reasonable basis to believe can be used to identify the individual. Thirteen individually identifiable health information components include many common identifiers (e.g., name, address, birth date, Social Security Number, etc.).

The Privacy Rule excludes from protected health information employment records that a covered entity maintains in its capacity as an employer and education and certain other records subject to, or defined in, the Family Educational Rights and Privacy Act (FERPA), 20 U.S.C. §1232g.

There are no restrictions on the use or disclosure of de-identified health information. De-identified health information neither identifies nor provides a reasonable basis to identify an individual. Two ways to de-identify information are a formal determination by a qualified statistician or the required removal of specified identifiers of the individual and of the individual's relatives, household members, and employers and is adequate only if the covered entity has no actual knowledge that the remaining information could be used to identify the individual.

A major purpose of the Privacy Rule is to define and limit the circumstances in which an individual's protected health information may be used, except either as the Privacy Rule permits or requires or as the individual who is the subject of the information (or the individual's personal representative) authorizes in writing.

A covered entity must disclose protected health information in only two situations: to individuals (or their personal representatives) specifically when they request access to or an accounting of disclosures of their protected health information and to HHS when it is undertaking a compliance investigation or review or enforcement action.

A covered entity is permitted, but not required, to use and disclose protected health information without an individual's authorization for the following purposes or situations:

- To the individual (unless required for access or accounting of disclosures);
- Treatment, Payment, and Health Care Operations (TPO);
- Opportunity to agree or object;
- Incident to an otherwise permitted use and disclosure;
- Public interest and benefit activities; and
- Limited data set for the purposes of research, public health, or health care operations.

In the second bullet above, Treatment, Payment, and Operations are defined as:

- **Treatment** is the provision, coordination, or management of health care and related services for an individual by one or more health care providers, including consultation between providers regarding a patient and referral of a patient by one provider to another.
- **Payment** encompasses the activities of a health plan to obtain premiums, determine or fulfill responsibilities for coverage and provision of benefits, and furnish or obtain reimbursement for health care delivered to an individual and activities of a health care provider to obtain payment or be reimbursed for the provision of health care to an individual.
- **Health care operations** are any of the following activities:
  ○ Quality assessment and improvement activities, including case management and care coordination;
  ○ Competency assurance activities, including provider or health plan performance evaluation, credentialing, and accreditation;
  ○ Conducting or arranging for medical reviews, audits, or legal services, including detection and compliance programs;
  ○ Specified insurance functions, such as underwriting, risk rating, and reinsuring risk;
  ○ Business planning, development, management, and administration; and
  ○ Business management and general administrative activities of the entity, including but not limited to de-identifying protected health information, creating a limited data set, and certain fundraising for the benefit of the covered entity and for those related to fraud and abuse.

Covered entities may rely on professional ethics and best judgments in deciding which of these permissive uses and disclosures to make:

- A covered entity may disclose protected health information to the individual who is the subject of the information.
- A covered entity may use and disclose protected health information for its own

treatment, payment, and health care operations activities. A covered entity also may disclose protected health information for the treatment activities of any health care provider, the payment activities of another covered entity and of any health care provider, or the health care operations of another covered entity involving either quality or competency assurance activities or fraud and abuse detection and compliance activities, if both covered entities have or had a relationship with the individual and the protected health information pertains to the relationship.

Audiologists may come in contact with psychiatric-related information. However, most uses and disclosures of psychotherapy notes for treatment, payment, and health care operations purposes require an authorization. While different, obtaining "consent" (written permission from individuals to use and disclose their protected health information for treatment, payment, and health care operations) is optional under the Privacy Rule for all covered entities. The content of a consent form, and the process for obtaining consent, are at the discretion of the covered entity electing to seek consent. Simply, authorizations are for specified purposes not otherwise allowed by the Privacy Rule and have an expiration date. Other requirements will be discussed in the next section.

Informal permission may be obtained by asking the individual outright, or by circumstances that clearly give the individual the opportunity to agree, acquiesce, or object. Where the individual is incapacitated as in an emergency situation or not available, covered entities generally may make such uses and disclosures if in the exercise of their professional judgment, the use or disclosure is determined to be in the best interests of the individual.

A covered entity also may rely on an individual's informal permission to disclose to the individual's family, relatives, or friends, or to other persons whom the individual identifies, protected health information directly relevant to that person's involvement in the individual's care or payment for care. For example, this provision allows an audiologist to discuss test results and recommendations to others acting on behalf of the patient. Similarly,

a covered entity may rely on an individual's informal permission to use or disclose protected health information for the purpose of notifying (including identifying or locating) family members, personal representatives, or others responsible for the individual's care of their general condition. In addition, protected health information may be disclosed for notification purposes to public or private entities authorized by law or charter.

The Privacy Rule does not require that every risk of an incidental use or disclosure of protected health information be eliminated. A use or disclosure of this information that occurs as a result of, or as "incident to," an otherwise permitted use or disclosure is permitted as long as the covered entity has adopted reasonable safeguards as required by the Privacy Rule, and the information being shared was limited to the "minimum necessary," also required by the Privacy Rule.

The Privacy Rule permits use and disclosure of protected health information without an individual's authorization or permission for 12 national priority purposes. These disclosures are permitted, although not required, by the Rule in recognition of the important uses made of health information outside of the health care context. Specific conditions or limitations apply to each public interest purpose, striking the balance between the individual privacy interest and the public interest need for this information.

Covered entities may disclose protected health information they believe is necessary to prevent or lessen a serious and imminent threat to a person or the public when such disclosure is made to someone they believe can prevent or lessen the threat, including the target of the threat. If the information is needed to identify or apprehend an escapee or violent criminal, covered entities may also disclose to law enforcement the information needed.

Authorization

An authorization is not required to use or disclose protected health information for certain essential government functions. Such functions include:

- Assuring proper execution of a military mission

- Conducting intelligence and national security activities that are authorized by law
- Providing protective services to the President
- Making medical suitability determinations for U.S. State Department employees
- Protecting the health and safety of inmates or employees in a correctional institution
- Determining eligibility for or conducting enrollment in certain government benefit programs

Covered entities may disclose protected health information as authorized by, and to comply with, Workers' Compensation laws and other similar programs providing benefits for work-related injuries or illnesses.

A limited data set is protected health information from which certain specified direct identifiers of individuals and their relatives, household members, and employers have been removed. A limited data set may be used and disclosed for research, health care operations, and public health purposes, provided the recipient enters into a data use agreement promising specified safeguards for the protected health information within the limited data set.

A covered entity must obtain the individual's written authorization for any use or disclosure of protected health information that is not for treatment, payment, or health care operations or otherwise permitted or required by the Privacy Rule. A covered entity may not condition treatment, payment, enrollment, or benefits eligibility on an individual granting an authorization, except in limited circumstances.

An authorization must be written in specific terms. It may allow use and disclosure of protected health information by the covered entity seeking the authorization, or by a third party. Examples of disclosures that would require an individual's authorization include:

- Disclosures to a life insurer for coverage purposes,
- Disclosures to an employer of the results of a pre-employment physical or lab test, or

- Disclosures to a pharmaceutical firm for their own marketing purposes.

All authorizations must be in plain language, and contain specific information regarding the information to be disclosed or used, the person(s) disclosing and receiving the information, the date of expiration, the right to revoke in writing, and other data. The Privacy Rule contains transition provisions applicable to authorizations and other express legal permissions obtained prior to April 14, 2003, the effective date.

A covered entity must obtain an individual's authorization to use or disclose psychotherapy notes with the following exceptions:

- Mandatory reporting of abuse.
- Mandatory requirement to warn someone if there are threats of "serious and imminent harm made by the patient." (State laws vary as to whether such a warning is mandatory or permissible.)
- For the lawful activities of a coroner or medical examiner or as required by law (CMS, 2014).

Marketing

Marketing is any communication about a product or service that encourages recipients to purchase or use the product or service. The Privacy Rule carves out the following health-related activities from this definition of marketing:

- "Pharmacies, health plans, and other covered entities must first obtain an individual's specific authorization before disclosing their patient information for marketing.
- At the same time, the rule permits doctors and other covered entities to communicate freely with patients about treatment options and other health-related information, including disease management programs.

Marketing also is an arrangement between a covered entity and any other entity whereby the covered entity discloses protected health information in exchange for direct or indirect remuneration or for the other entity to communicate about its own products or services encouraging the use or purchase of those products or services. A covered entity must obtain an authorization to use or disclose protected health information for marketing, except for face-to-face marketing, communications between a covered entity and an individual, and for a covered entity's provision of promotional gifts of nominal value. No authorization is needed, however, to make a communication that falls within one of the exceptions to the marketing definition. An authorization for marketing that involves the covered entity's receipt of direct or indirect remuneration from a third party must reveal that fact.

"Minimum Necessary"

A central aspect of the Privacy Rule is the principle of "minimum necessary" use and disclosure. A covered entity must make reasonable efforts to use, disclose, and request only the minimum amount of protected health information needed to accomplish the intended purpose of the use, disclosure, or request. A covered entity must develop and implement policies and procedures to reasonably limit uses and disclosures to the minimum necessary. When the minimum necessary standard applies to a use or disclosure, a covered entity may not use, disclose, or request the entire medical record for a particular purpose, unless it can specifically justify the whole record as the amount reasonably needed for the purpose.

The minimum necessary requirement is not imposed in any of the following circumstances:

- Disclosure to or a request by a health care provider for treatment;
- Disclosure to an individual who is the subject of the information, or the individual's personal representative;
- Use or disclosure made pursuant to an authorization;
- Disclosure to HHS for complaint investigation, compliance review, or enforcement;

- Use or disclosure that is required by law; or
- Use or disclosure required for compliance with the HIPAA Transactions Rule or other HIPAA Administrative Simplification Rules.

For internal use, a covered entity must develop and implement policies and procedures that restrict access and use of protected health information based on the specific roles of the members of their facility. These policies and procedures must identify the persons, or classes of persons, in their setting who need access to protected health information to carry out their duties, the categories of protected health information to which access is needed, and any conditions under which they need the information to do their jobs.

Covered entities must establish and implement policies and procedures (which may be standard protocols) for routine, recurring disclosures, or requests for disclosures, that limit the protected health information disclosed to that which is the minimum amount reasonably necessary to achieve the purpose of the disclosure. Individual review of each disclosure is not required. For non-routine, non-recurring disclosures, or requests for disclosures that it makes, covered entities must develop criteria designed to limit disclosures to the information reasonably necessary to accomplish the purpose of the disclosure and review each of these requests individually in accordance with the established criteria. If another covered entity makes a request for protected health information, a covered entity may rely, if reasonable under the circumstances, on the request as complying with this minimum necessary standard. Similarly, a covered entity may rely on requests as being the minimum necessary protected health information from:

- A public official;
- A professional (such as an attorney or accountant) who is the covered entity's business associate, seeking the information to provide services to or for the covered entity; or
- A researcher who provides the documentation or representation required by the Privacy Rule for research.

Notice of Privacy Practices (NPP)

Each covered entity, with certain exceptions, must provide a notice of its privacy practices (NPP). The Privacy Rule requires that the notice contain certain elements and must describe the ways in which the covered entity may use and disclose protected health information. The notice must state the covered entity's duties to protect privacy, provide a notice of privacy practices, and abide by the terms of the current notice. The notice must describe individuals' rights, including the right to complain to HHS and to the covered entity if they believe their privacy rights have been violated. The notice must include a point of contact for the designated privacy officer for further information and for making complaints to the covered entity. Covered entities must act in accordance with their notices. The rule also contains specific distribution requirements for direct treatment providers, all other health care providers, and health plans.

A covered health care provider with a direct treatment relationship with individuals must deliver a privacy practices notice to patients as follows:

- Not later than the first service encounter by personal delivery (for patient visits), by automatic and contemporaneous electronic response (for electronic service delivery), and by prompt mailing (for telephonic service delivery);
- By posting the notice at each service delivery site in a clear and prominent place where people seeking service may reasonably be expected to be able to read the notice; and
- In emergency treatment situations, the provider must furnish its notice as soon as practicable after the emergency abates.

Covered entities, whether direct treatment providers or indirect treatment providers (including audiologists) or health plans must supply notice to anyone on request. A covered entity must also make its notice electronically available on any web site it maintains for customer service or benefits information. The covered entities in an organized health care arrangement may use a joint privacy practices notice, as long as each agrees to abide by the notice content with respect to the protected health information created by or received in connection with participation in the arrangement. Distribution of a joint notice by any covered entity participating in an Organized Health Care Arrangement (OHCA) at the first point that an OHCA member has an obligation to provide notice satisfies the distribution obligation of the other participants in the OHCA. A health plan must distribute its privacy practices notice to each of its enrollees by its Privacy Rule compliance date. Thereafter, the health plan must give its notice to each new enrollee at enrollment, and send a reminder to every enrollee at least once every three years that the notice is available on request. A health plan satisfies its distribution obligation by furnishing the notice to the "named insured," that is, the subscriber for coverage that also applies to spouses and dependents.

A covered health care provider with a direct treatment relationship with individuals must make a good faith effort to obtain written acknowledgment from patients of receipt of the privacy practices notice and is relieved of the need to request acknowledgment in an emergency treatment. The provider must document the reason for any failure to obtain the patient's written acknowledgment; the Privacy Rule does not prescribe any particular content for the acknowledgment. Except in certain circumstances, individuals have the right to review and obtain a copy of their protected health information in a covered entity's designated record set. The "designated record set" is that group of records maintained by or for a covered entity that is used, in whole or part, to make decisions about individuals, or that is a provider's medical and billing records about individuals or a health plan's enrollment, payment, claims adjudication, and case or medical management record systems. The Rule contains exceptions from the right of access of the following protected health information:

- Psychotherapy notes.
- Information compiled for legal proceedings.
- Laboratory results to which the Clinical Laboratory Improvement Act (CLIA) prohibits access, or information held by certain research laboratories.

For information included within the right of access, covered entities may deny an individual access in certain specified situations, such as when an audiologist believes access could cause harm to the individual or another. In such situations, the individual must be given the right to have such denials reviewed by a licensed clinical audiologist for a second opinion. Covered entities may impose reasonable, cost-based fees for the cost of copying and postage.

Amending Protected Health Information (PHI)

The Rule gives individuals the right to have covered entities amend their protected health information in a designated record set when that information is inaccurate or incomplete. If a covered entity accepts an amendment request, it must make reasonable efforts to provide the amendment to persons that the individual has identified as needing it and to persons that the covered entity knows might rely on the information to the individual's detriment. If the request is denied, covered entities must provide the individual with a written denial and allow the individual to submit a statement of disagreement for inclusion in the record. The Rule specifies processes for requesting and responding to a request for amendment. A covered entity must amend protected health information in its designated record set on receipt of notice to amend from another covered entity.

Disclosures

Individuals have a right to an accounting of the disclosures of their protected health information by a covered entity or the covered entity's business associates. The maximum disclosure accounting period is the six years immediately preceding the accounting request, except a covered entity is not obligated to account for any disclosure made before its Privacy Rule compliance date. The Privacy Rule does not require accounting for disclosures:

- For treatment, payment, or health care operations;
- To the individual or the individual's personal representative;

- For notification of or to persons involved in an individual's health care or payment for health care, for disaster relief, or for facility directories;
- Pursuant to an authorization;
- Of a limited data set;
- For national security or intelligence purposes;
- To correctional institutions or law enforcement officials for certain purposes regarding inmates or individuals in lawful custody; or
- Incident to otherwise permitted or required uses or disclosures. Accounting for disclosures to health oversight agencies and law enforcement officials must be temporarily suspended on their written representation that an accounting would likely impede their activities.

Individuals have the right to request that a covered entity restrict use or disclosure of protected health information for treatment, payment, or health care operations, disclosure to persons involved in the individual's health care or payment for health care, or disclosure to notify family members or others about the individual's general condition, location, or death. A covered entity is under no obligation to agree to requests for restrictions. A covered entity that does agree must comply with the agreed upon restrictions, except for purposes of treating the individual in a medical emergency.

Health plans and covered health care providers must permit individuals to request an alternative means or location for receiving communications of protected health information by means other than those the covered entity typically employs. For example, an individual may request the provider communicate with the individual through a designated address or phone number. Similarly, an individual may request the provider send communications in a closed envelope rather than a post card. Health plans must accommodate reasonable requests if the individual indicates that the disclosure of all or part of the protected health information could endanger the individual and may not question the individual's statement of endangerment. Any covered entity may condition compliance with a confidential communication request on the individual specifying an alternative address or method of contact and explaining how any payment will be handled.

HHS recognizes that covered entities range from the smallest provider to the largest, multistate health plan. Therefore, the flexibility and scalability of the Rule are intended to allow covered entities to analyze their own needs and implement solutions appropriate for their own environment. What is appropriate for a particular covered entity will depend on the nature of the covered entity's business, as well as the covered entity's size and resources.

Privacy Policies and Compliance Officer

A covered entity must develop and implement written privacy policies and procedures that are consistent with the Privacy Rule. A covered entity must designate a privacy official responsible for developing and implementing its privacy policies and procedures and a contact person or contact office responsible for receiving complaints and providing individuals with information on the covered entity's privacy practices.

Workforce members include employees, volunteers, trainees, and may also include other persons whose conduct is under the direct control of the entity (whether they are paid by the entity). A covered entity must train all workforce members on its privacy policies and procedures as necessary and appropriate for them to carry out their functions. A covered entity must have and apply appropriate sanctions against workforce members who violate its privacy policies and procedures or the Privacy Rule. A covered entity must mitigate to the extent practicable, any harmful effects it learns was caused by use or disclosure of protected health information by its workforce or its business associates in violation of its privacy policies and procedures or the Privacy Rule.

Safeguards

A covered entity must maintain reasonable and appropriate administrative, technical, and physi-

cal safeguards to prevent intentional or unintentional use or disclosure of protected health information in violation of the Privacy Rule and to limit its incidental use and disclosure pursuant to otherwise permitted or required use or disclosure. For example, such safeguards might include shredding documents containing protected health information before discarding them, securing medical records with lock and key or passcode, and limiting access to keys or passcodes.

Complaints

A covered entity must have procedures for individuals to complain about its compliance with its privacy policies and procedures and the Privacy Rule. The covered entity must explain those procedures in its Notice of Privacy Practices (NPP). Among other things, the covered entity must identify individuals to whom one can submit complaints (privacy officer) and advise that complaints can be submitted to the covered entity and to the Secretary of HHS.

A covered entity may not retaliate against a person for exercising rights provided by the Privacy Rule, for assisting in an investigation by HHS or another appropriate authority, or for opposing an act or practice that the person believes in good faith violates the Privacy Rule. A covered entity may not require an individual to waive any right under the Privacy Rule as a condition for obtaining treatment, payment, and enrollment or benefits eligibility.

A covered entity must maintain its privacy policies and procedures, its privacy practices notices, disposition of complaints and other actions, activities, and designations that the Privacy Rule requires to be documented until six years after the later of the date of their creation or last effective date.

The only administrative obligations which a fully insured group health plan that has no more than enrollment data and summary health information is required to comply with are the ban on retaliatory acts and the waiver of individual rights and documentation requirements with respect to plan documents if such documents are amended to provide for the disclosure of protected health information to the plan sponsor by a health insurance issuer or HMO that services the group health plan.

State laws that are contrary to the Privacy Rule are preempted by the federal requirements, whereby the federal requirements will apply. "Contrary" means that it would be impossible for a covered entity to comply with both the state and federal requirements, or that the provision of state law is an obstacle to accomplishing the full purposes and objectives of the Administrative Simplification provisions of HIPAA. The Privacy Rule provides exceptions to the general rule of federal preemption for contrary state laws that relate to the privacy of individually identifiable health information and provide greater privacy protections or privacy rights with respect to such information as well as provide for the reporting of disease, injury, child abuse, birth, death, public health surveillance, investigation, intervention, or certain health plan reporting, such as for management or financial audits.

Consistent with the principles for achieving compliance provided in the Rule, HHS will seek the cooperation of covered entities and may provide technical assistance to help them comply voluntarily with the Rule. The Rule provides processes for persons to file complaints with HHS, describes the responsibilities of covered entities to provide records and compliance reports, and to cooperate with and permit access to information for investigations and compliance reviews.

Penalties

HHS may impose civil money penalties on a covered entity of $100 per failure to comply with a Privacy Rule requirement and may not exceed $25,000 per year for multiple violations of the identical Privacy Rule requirement in a calendar year. HHS may not impose a civil money penalty under specific circumstances, such as when a violation is due to reasonable cause and did not involve willful neglect and the covered entity corrected the violation within 30 days of when it knew or should have known of the violation.

A person who knowingly obtains or discloses individually identifiable health information in violation of HIPAA faces a fine of $50,000 and up to one year imprisonment. The criminal penalties increase to $100,000 and up to five year's imprisonment if the wrongful conduct involves false pretenses, and to $250,000 and up to ten year's imprisonment if the wrongful conduct involves the intent to sell, transfer, or use individually identifiable health information for commercial advantage, personal gain, or malicious harm. Criminal sanctions will be enforced by the Department of Justice.

HIPAA Security

Prior to HIPAA, no generally accepted set of security standards or general requirements for protecting health information existed in the health care industry. At the same time, new technologies were evolving and the health care industry began to move away from paper processes and rely more heavily on the use of electronic information systems to pay claims, answer eligibility questions, provide health information, and conduct a host of other administrative and clinically based functions. Today, audiologists are using clinical applications such as electronic health records (EHR) and electronic billing systems. Health plans are providing access to claims and care management as well as subscriber/member self-service applications. While this means that the health care workforce, and in particular audiologists, can be more mobile and efficient (i.e., audiologists can check patient records and test results from wherever they are located as well as the ongoing advancement into telemedicine and/or tele-audiology), the rise in the adoption rate of these technologies increases potential security risks. A major goal of the Security Rule is to protect the privacy of individuals' health information while allowing covered entities to adopt new technologies to improve the quality and efficiency of patient care while assuring the confidentiality, integrity, and availability of e-PHI (electronic Personal Health Information). Given that the health care marketplace is diverse, the Security Rule is designed to be flexible and scalable so a covered entity can implement policies, procedures, and technologies that are appropriate for the entity's particular size, organizational structure, and risks to consumers' e-PHI. The Security

Rule does not apply to PHI transmitted orally or in writing.

HIPAA Security Rule Requirements

The Security Rule requires covered entities to maintain reasonable and appropriate administrative, technical, and physical safeguards for protecting PHI. Specifically, covered entities must:

- Ensure the confidentiality, integrity, and availability of all PHI, electronic and hard copy, created, received, maintained, or transmitted;
- Identify and protect against reasonably anticipated threats to the security or integrity of the information;
- Protect against reasonably anticipated, impermissible uses or disclosures; and
- Ensure compliance by their workforce

Confidentiality

The Security Rule defines "confidentiality" to mean that PHI is not available or disclosed to unauthorized persons. The Security Rule's confidentiality requirements support the Privacy Rule's prohibitions against improper uses and disclosures of PHI. The Security Rule also promotes the two additional goals of maintaining the integrity and availability of PHI. Under the Security Rule, "Integrity" means that PHI is not altered or destroyed in an unauthorized manner. "Availability" means that PHI is accessible and usable on demand by an authorized person. HHS recognizes that covered entities range from the smallest provider to the largest, multi-state health plan. Therefore, the Security Rule is flexible and scalable to allow covered entities to analyze their own needs and implement solutions appropriate for their specific environments. What is appropriate for a particular covered entity will depend on the nature of the covered entity's business, as well as the covered entity's size and resources. Covered entities must review and modify their security measures to continue protecting PHI in a changing environment.

Risk Analysis

The Administrative Safeguards provisions in the Security Rule require covered entities to perform risk analysis as part of their security management processes. The risk analysis and management provisions of the Security Rule include analysis of security management processes, security personnel, information access management, workforce training and management, and evaluation. Physical safeguards must address facility access and control, and workstation and device security. Technical safeguards must address access control, audit controls, integrity controls, and transmission security.

A risk analysis process includes, but is not limited to, the following activities:

- Evaluate the likelihood and impact of potential risks to PHI;
- Implement appropriate security measures to address the risks identified in the risk analysis;
- Document the chosen security measures and, where required, the rationale for adopting those measures; and
- Maintain continuous, reasonable, and appropriate security protections.

Risk analysis should be an ongoing process, in which a covered entity regularly reviews its records to track access to PHI and detect security incidents, periodically evaluates the effectiveness of security measures put in place, and regularly reevaluates potential risks to PHI.

If a covered entity knows of an activity or practice of the business associate that constitutes a material breach or violation of the business associate's obligation, the covered entity must take reasonable steps to cure the breach or end the violation. Violations include the failure to implement safeguards that reasonably and appropriately protect PHI. A covered entity must adopt reasonable and appropriate policies and procedures to comply with the provisions of the Security Rule. A covered entity must maintain written security assessments for six years after the latter of the date of their creation or last effective date.

In general, state laws that are contrary to the HIPAA regulations are preempted by the federal requirements, meaning that the federal requirements will apply. "Contrary" means that it would be impossible for a covered entity to comply with both the state and federal requirements, or that the provision of state law is an obstacle in accomplishing the full purposes and objectives of the administrative simplification provisions of HIPAA.

Final Thoughts

This goal of this chapter was to highlight the ongoing interaction and potentially the inevitable collision between issues involving the legal arena and the practice of audiology. This area will continue to evolve and there is little doubt that further case and legislative law will come forth that may impact audiologists and the many internal and external stakeholders including patients, organizations, manufacturers, and, of course, the legal arena, among others. This evolution hopefully will spawn greater efforts into educating all stakeholders regarding the potential legal, ethical, technological, economic, financial, and risk management impacts within our profession. Ignorance of the potential legal and social ramifications will not be a valid defense for improper or inappropriate behavior nor should it. It will behoove all stakeholders to recognize and accept their responsibilities and adopt any and all relevant legal and risk mitigation strategies when functioning within the scope of practice of the profession and in all of their interactions with other stakeholders.

References

Black, H. (1990). *Black's Law Dictionary*. St. Paul, MN: West Publishing Company.

Bricker and Eckler, LLP. (2010). Overpayments—the clock is ticking to report and return that money, *Health Care Reform Express*, June 1–2. Retrieved July 12, 2015 from www.brickler.com.

Centers for Medicare and Medicaid Services, Department of Health and Human Services, Office of the Inspector General. 42 CFR Part 1001. (1991). Retrieved March 30, 2016 from http://oig.hhs.gov/fraud/docs/safeharborregulations/072991.htm.

Centers for Medicare and Medicaid Services, Department of Health and Human Services. (2011). The Medicare Overpayment Collection Process: Fact Sheet. ICN006379. Retrieved July 12, 2015 from www.cms.gov.

Centers for Medicare and Medicaid Services. (2014). HIPAA Privacy Rule and Sharing Information Related to Mental Health. Retrieved March 23, 2016 from http://www.hhs.gov/hipaa/for-professionals/special-topics/mental-health/index.html.

Centers for Medicare and Medicaid Services. (2016). HIPAA Privacy Rules. Retrieved on March 23, 2016 from http://www.cms.k12.nc.us/Jobs/benefits/health/Pages/HIPAA.aspx.

Centers for Medicare and Medicaid Services United States Government Accountability Office. (2012). Report to Congressional Requesters. Medicare Implementation and Financial Incentive Programs Under Federal Fraud and Abuse Laws. Retrieved March 1, 2016 from http://gao.gov/assets/590/589793.pdf.

Foltner, K. and Lewis, D. (2007). Risks, rewards, retribution. *Advance for Hearing Practice Management*. 9(3):30.

Grant, D. and Kyles, J. (2013). *Fraud and Abuse Answer Book, Medicare Compliance Alert*. Rockville, MD: Decision Health.

Health Insurance Portability and Accountability Act of 1996 Pub. Law 104-191, 45 CFR 160-164. Retrieved July 14, 2015 from https://aspe.hhs.gov/report/standards-privacy-individually-identifiable-health-information-regulation-text.

HealthReform.Gov. Retrieved July 14, 2015 from http://kff.org/health-reform/fact-sheet/summary-of-the-affordable-care-act/.

Lewis, D. (2012). An overview of the Federal False Claims Act, *Audiology Today*. 24, 55–58.

Lewis, D. (2012). Anti-kickback considerations for the hearing healthcare practitioner. *The Hearing Professional*. 1, 28–31.

Lewis, D. (2005). A small rural hospital's corporate compliance program and its recipe for success in a highly regulated and scrutinized business environment. Doctoral Dissertation. Kennedy Western University Program, Library of Congress.

Lupe, Mark. (2003). The anti-kickback prohibition, University of Missouri Health Care Presentation.

Raspant M. and Auten, M. (2011). Why is qui tam litigation so difficult to resolve? *AHLA Connections*. 22–27.

U.S. Department of Health and Human Services Office of Inspector General. (2014). A Roadmap for new physicians: Avoiding Medicare and Medicaid fraud and abuse. Retrieved July 7, 2015 from https://oig.hhs.gov/compliance/physician-education/roadmap_web_version.pdf.

Warren Benson Law Group. (2011). Los Angeles, CA. Retrieved July 7, 2015 from http://www.warrenbensonlaw.com.

ZPIC Audit. (2010). Number of false claims act investigations being pursued is currently at an all time high . . . and is likely to go even higher due to changes to the False Claims Act under health care reform. Retrieved July 7, 2015 from http://zpicaudit.com/tag/false-claims-act/.

CHAPTER 4

Third-Party Reimbursement, Contracting, and Credentialing for Audiology Services

Kimberly M. Cavitt

Introduction

In the United States, third-party reimbursement is defined as "reimbursement for services rendered to a person in whom an entity other than the receiver of the service is responsible for the payment" (Mosby, 2009). Third-party reimbursement typically comes in the form of coverage, in whole or in part, from entities such as:

- Health insurance plans
- Early intervention and children's disability programs
- State and federal worker's compensation plans and programs
- Veteran's Administration
- Third-party administrators

Health Insurance Plans

Health insurance plans are payers, either funded, subsidized, and offered by the insured's employer, subsidized by state or federal entities, or purchased by an individual who for a monthly fee, cover an individual patient's approved medical and surgical health care costs. Some common examples of health insurance plans are:

- Medicare: A federal health insurance program for those who are 65 or older, certain younger people with specific disabilities, and those with End-Stage Renal Disease (ESRD) for those who have permanent kidney failure requiring dialysis or a transplant (Medicare, 2015).
- Medicaid: A joint federal and state program that assists low-income individuals or families to pay for the costs associated with long-term medical and custodial care provided they financially qualify. Although the federal government largely funds Medicaid, it is administered by each state and coverage and benefits vary (Investopedia, 2005).
- Private insurance carriers: These entities are funded and/or subsidized by an employer and/or an individual to provide coverage and benefits for allowed medical and surgical conditions. Some common examples are BlueCross/BlueShield, United Healthcare, Cigna, Aetna, Humana, and Kaiser Permanente.

Early Intervention and Children's Disability Programs

Early intervention and children's disability programs are typically federal and state programs that provide medical, educational support, and funding of specialized educational and health care services to children three years of age or younger who are at increased risk for medical and/or educational delays or challenges.

State and Federal Workers' Compensations Programs

State and federal workers' compensation programs offer employer covered insurance and compensation in order to provide coverage and benefits to employees who become injured on the job. Through these programs, workers can be provided with monetary compensation and health care for the remainder of their lives.

Veteran's Administration

The Veteran's Administration (VA) is a workers' compensation and health care system, as well as a form of health insurance for veterans of the U.S. armed forces. This program is administered by the U.S. Department of Veteran's Affairs through its federally operated hospitals and clinics. Some VA hospitals outsource health care to non-VA providers in the private sector through their contract services or fee basis programs.

Third-Party Administrators

Third-party administrators are companies or insurance plans that provide coverage and benefits, discount programs, cost containment, claims processing, and/or claims management for another insurance entity or employer. Some common third-party administrators in hearing health care are EPIC, Amplifon Hearing, HearUSA, Tru-Hearing, and American Hearing Benefits.

Insurance Terminology

- Accountable Care Organization (ACO): Groups of physicians, hospitals, and other health care providers, who voluntarily join to provide coordinated high-quality care to their traditional Medicare patients. The goal of this coordinated care is to ensure that patients, especially the chronically ill, receive the appropriate care at the appropriate time, while avoiding unnecessary duplication of services and preventing medical errors. When an ACO succeeds in delivering high-quality care and reducing costs, it will share in the savings it achieves for the Medicare program with the ACO itself (Centers for Medicare and Medicaid Services, 2015).
- Allowed Charge (approved charge, allowable): Payment for an item or service under the customary and current system outlined on the payer fee schedule; inclusive of the payment from the primary payer, the secondary payer, the deductible, the co-pay, and/or the co-insurance.
- Appeal: A request for a health insurer or plan to review a previous coverage decision or payment and make an amended determination of coverage or denial.
- Assignment of Benefits: A procedure where the member/beneficiary authorizes the payer to make payment of allowable benefits directly to the rendering provider.
- Bad Debt: The amount that a practice must write off due to a patient's failure to meet their financial responsibilities.
- Balance Billing: Billing the patient for any amount in excess of the allowed by the payer; billing the difference between what the payer allows and the provider's usual and customary rate to the patient.
- Beneficiary: A person eligible to receive benefits under a health plan; the insured.
- Benefits: The health care items or services covered under a health insurance plan.
- Billed Charges: The amount the provider bills to the payer for a specific item or service; same as "submitted charges."

- Carrier: The insurance company that writes and administers the health insurance policy; the payer.
- Carve Out: Where an item or service or groups of items are not covered in a health insurance contract between the payer and the provider as they are usually reimbursed according to a different payment arrangement or rate formula than those services (Mosby, 2015).
- Clean Claim: A claim submitted to the payer that includes all the required information and lacks any complications that might cause delays in payment processing and payment (Medical Dictionary for the Health Professions and Nursing, 2015).
- Co-insurance: A provision of an insurance plan by which the beneficiary shares in the cost of certain covered expenses with the payer on a percentage basis; cost-sharing.
- Coordination of Benefits: A provision in an insurance plan that, when a patient has coverage by multiple insurance plans, benefits paid by all the plans will never exceed 100% of the total claim.
- Co-payment: The provision of an insurance plan by which the beneficiary is required to pay a fixed portion of the cost of their healthcare expenses. This is typically a per visit fee and is often printed directly on the patient's insurance card.
- Contractual Adjustment: The difference between a provider's usual and customary fee and the amount allowed by the payer; same as a "write-off."
- Council of Affordable Quality Healthcare (CAQH): A non-profit organization that collaborates with healthcare providers, trade associations, and insurers to provide centralized credentialing services and healthcare initiatives (CAQH, 2015).
- Credentialing: The process by which third-party payers determine that a facility and/or a provider are qualified to see their members for the provision of healthcare items and services (Aetna, 2015).
- Customary Charge: The provider's standard charge for a given item or service.

- Date of Service: The date the service is performed or the item is dispensed.
- Discount Benefit: This is where a third party negotiates unfunded discounts for specific items or services on behalf of their members.
- Deductible: A stipulated annual amount which the beneficiary must pay toward the cost of their health care before the benefits and coverage of the plan go into effect; usually a set dollar amount that must be satisfied within a given calendar year.
- Direct Supervision: In an outpatient setting, direct supervision is when the physician or non-physician practitioner is "immediately available" or "physically present, interruptible and able to furnish assistance and direction throughout the performance of the procedure"; the physician or non-physician practitioner does not have to be present in the same room when the procedure is being performed (Hallrender, 2015).
- Durable Medical Equipment (DME): Equipment, items, goods, and supplies ordered by a health care provider for everyday or extended use; a cochlear implant, an osseo-integrated device, and a hearing aid are considered to be DME by some payers.
- Electronic Medical Record (EMR): A computerized, digitally stored and transmitted medical record, often referred to as an Electronic Health Record (EHR).
- Eligible Expenses: Same as "allowable" and "negotiated rate."
- Explanation of Benefits (EOB): A form included with your payment/denial from the payer in which the payer explains the specifics of coverage, denial, and/or payment for a specific patient for a given date of service; it also outlines the patient's financial responsibilities.
- Excluded services: Health care items and services that a health insurance plan doesn't pay for or cover; same as "non-covered service."
- Exclusions: Specific services or conditions which the insurance policy will not cover or which are covered at a limited rate.

- Fee for Service: Refers to reimbursing health care providers for the individual items and services provided.
- Funded Benefit: A benefit for a specific item or service that is paid in whole or in part by a third-party payer.
- General supervision: An item or service is furnished under the overall direction and control of the supervising physician or non-physician practitioner, but his or her physical presence is not required during the dispensing of the item or the performance of the procedure (Hallrender, 2015).
- Health Maintenance Organization (HMO): Type of insurance plan which represents "pre-paid" or "capitated" insurance plans in which individuals or their employers pay a fixed monthly fee for services instead of a separate charge for each visit or service. The monthly fees remain the same, regardless of types or levels of services provided and are provided by physicians who are employed by, or under contract with, the HMO (Health Insurance, 2015). Many HMO members do not have coverage and benefits when they see providers outside of the HMO network.
- Incident to: Defined as services or supplies furnished as an integral, although incidental, part of the physician's personal professional services in the course of diagnosis or treatment of an injury or illness. These services are furnished under the supervision of the attending physician and, as a result, billed under the NPI of this physician as the rendering provider (Incident to Services, 2015).
- In-Network (participating): The provider has been credentialed by a specific payer and has agreed to the terms of their payer agreement/contract; the provider must typically accept the allowable as payment in full when they are in-network.
- Insurance Mandates: When a state specifically mandates that specific insurers in their state cover specific items and services. For example, at the time of publication, 20 states had mandates for hearing aid coverage (AG Bell, 2015).
- Insured: The individual who represents the family unit in relation to the insurance benefits and coverage; usually the employee who holds the insurance provided by their employer and may include their dependents.
- Insurer: Payer.
- Medically Reasonable and Necessary: Health care services, items, or supplies needed to prevent, diagnose, or treat an illness, injury, condition, disease, or its symptoms and that meet accepted standards of medicine.
- Member: Same as "beneficiary."
- Negotiated Rate: Same as "allowable" and "eligible expenses."
- Network: The facilities, providers, and suppliers a health insurer or plan has contracted with to provide health care services and care.
- Non-Covered Service: An item or service that is not a covered benefit under a specific insurance plan; same as "excluded services."
- Order: A request from one healthcare provider to another healthcare provider requesting that they perform a specific item or service to a given patient; same as "referral" or "prior authorization."
- Out of Pocket Expense: Limitation on the amount a beneficiary must personally contribute to their healthcare costs in a given year; can affect co-insurance.
- Out-of-Network: The provider has not been credentialed by a specific payer and has not agreed to accept the terms of the payer agreement/contract; can bill the patient your usual and customary rate; patient's coverage and benefits often reduced or non-existent.
- Patient Responsibility: The amount the patient owes for a given item or service once the payer has processed the claim.
- Payable Amount: The amount paid by the payer for a given item or service; excludes co-insurance, co-payments, and deductibles.
- Personal supervision: The physician or non-physician practitioner is present, for

the entire patient visit, in the room when the item is being dispensed or the service is being performed (Hallrender, 2015).

- Point of Service (POS) plan: This is a type of managed care plan that is a hybrid of HMO and PPO plans. Like an HMO, participants designate an in-network physician to be their primary care provider, and like a PPO, members may see providers outside of the POS network for health care services. When members see out of network providers, they typically have more out of pocket costs for the care they receive unless they are specifically referred to an out of network provider (Healthcare Coverage Guide, 2015).

- Predetermination: The process of obtaining a written estimate of what a payer will pay for specific items and services before the item is dispensed or the service is performed; predeterminations are not a guarantee of payment.

- Preferred Provider Organization (PPO): This is a managed, health insurance plan where health care providers and facilities contractually agree with an insurer to provide medical and surgical care to that insurer's members at a reduced reimbursement rate. Members of a PPO typically have more flexibility with the providers they can choose to see. If the provider is in the PPO network, coverage and benefits are typically more advantageous than if they see a provider who is not part of the PPO network.

- Primary Insurance: The payer who has the primary responsibility for payment under the coordination of benefits provisions of the patient's insurance agreement.

- Prior Authorization: A requirement by the payer that coverage for a given item or service is dependent on the item or service being approved by the payer or another health care entity before the item or service is provided to the beneficiary.

- Provider: The individual who provides items and services to beneficiaries.

- Referral: Same as "order."

- Secondary Insurance: The payer who has the secondary responsibility for payment under the coordination of benefits provisions of the patient's insurance agreement.

- Submitted Charges: Same as "billed charges."

- Usual and Customary Fees: A practices' fee for a given item or service, regardless of payer.

- Utilization Review: The process of reviewing items and services provided by a specific provider or facility to determine if the items and services provided were reasonable and necessary; a provision included in most third-party contracts.

- Verification: The act of predetermining eligibility, coverage, and benefits for a specific patient for specific items and services; verifications of benefits are not a guarantee of payment.

- Write-Offs: The amount that is not paid by the payer but cannot be billed to the beneficiary; same as "contractual adjustment."

The Who, What, and Where of Third-Party Contracting

Other than traditional Medicare, audiologists are typically voluntary participants in the third-party arena. In other words, audiology practices and their providers do not have to enroll as in-network providers with specific third-party insurers. Many audiologists can and do decide to be out of network providers. Patients should just be informed of a facility's third-party participation status prior to scheduling an appointment as the patient's financial responsibilities can and will be affected.

If an audiology practice decides to explore enrollment in a third-party plan, it should begin by gathering information about the payer and their enrollment processes. Practices first need to determine which third-party payers they are interested in potentially contracting with for covered services by doing a market analysis of their community. This can be accomplished by gaining answers to these questions:

1. What insurers represent or provide coverage for the major employers in the practice's community?
2. What insurance plans do referring and ordering physicians and local hospitals accept?
3. What insurers offer lucrative reimbursement, specifically for hearing aids?

The answers to these questions can guide a practice in determining which third-party payers in their area should be explored for potential enrollment as an in-network provider. The best means of beginning this evaluation and enrollment process is to consult the payer website, found with an Internet search of the payer name and your state. For example, to locate information about BlueCross/BlueShield of Illinois, one would search "Illinois BlueCross/Blue Shield." Once the website is located, the practice owner and/or manager should review the resources available in the "provider" section of the website. Many payers have detailed information about their enrollment procedures, policies, guidelines, and requirements and are just as vital to review as the contractual agreement itself. In many cases, the enrollment process can be initiated from this section of the payers' website.

Enrollment

Before an audiologist or practice can consider enrollment as an in-network provider with a third-party payer, they need, at a minimum, to be able to provide the following information:

- Business name
- Employer Identification Number (EIN) from the Internal Revenue Service (IRS)
- Organization or facility National Provider Identifier (NPI)
- Business address
- Liability insurance for the business and each provider

- State audiology and/or hearing aid license number for each provider of care
- NPI for each provider of care

Once your application/enrollment request has been received and processed by a given third-party payer, the facility or provider will receive correspondence from the payer and can take one of the following forms:

- The third-party payer may send the facility or provider a rejection letter. Third-party payers can and do say no to enrolling new facilities and providers into their network. In this situation, the payers' provider network may be full and they are not accepting new providers into their audiology network.
- The third-party payer may send the facility or provider an enrollment/contractual agreement and a fee schedule of allowable charges.

If the third-party payer rejects a business' enrollment and participation in their provider network would be lucrative for that business, it is recommended that the facility complete one of the following actions:

- Periodically attempt to re-enroll with the payer.
- Contact the employer's human resources department that provides coverage and benefits to their employees through this third-party payer.
- Have affected patients contact the payer and/or the human resources department of their employer and request that the facility and its providers be considered for inclusion in the network.
- Purchase another audiology, vestibular, and/or hearing aid practice that is currently an in-network provider for this payer.

It is important that the denied facility have data to illustrate how many of the third-party payers members are seeking their services as an out-of-network provider, how underserved the community is (if a patient has to drive more than 5 miles to see an in-network provider) in terms of audiology and vestibular services, and/or how this specific audiology practice offers services or products not provided by other in-network providers (such as auditory processing, vestibular or tinnitus evaluation or management, pediatrics, or implants).

If the third-party payer sends the facility and its providers a contractual agreement to review and complete, it is important that a representative of the practice make a copy of the agreement for their records, read the entire agreement, and pose questions to the third-party payer when clarification is warranted or questions need to be addressed. It is strongly recommended that audiologists seek the advice of legal counsel prior to signing any contractual agreements.

Contract Review Considerations

Some important considerations audiology practices need to address when evaluating a third-party agreement include, but are not limited to:

- If the practice signs this participation agreement, what insurance products would they be participating with? In other words, would they be required to participate with the payer's Medicare Part C (Medicare Advantage) program? Their privatized, managed Medicaid program? Their HMO or ACO product offerings? What, if any, are the specific requirements that are unique to each insurance product offering? Does each product have its own fee schedule?
- Does the plan allow for patients to upgrade their hearing aids to something more expensive or advanced than that allowed by the allowable rate? In other words, can the patient be financially responsible for the difference between the payers' allowable rate for the hearing aid related services and the practices' usual and customary fee for a more expensive or advanced device? If the plan does allow for patient upgrades, what is the process of patient notification

and authorization of the accompanying financial responsibilities?
- Does it require patients to complete notices of non-coverage before non-covered services are provided?
- Can student externs, audiology assistants, or technicians see members of the plan? If yes, are there supervision requirements and, if so, what are those requirements?
- Can licensed hearing aid dispensers see members of the plan? If yes, for what covered services?
- Can certain items or services be carved out of the contract?
- Does the agreement automatically renew or "evergreen" each year on the anniversary of the effective date? If not, what are the renewal terms?
- What are the terms under which either party can terminate the agreement?
- What are the terms under which the agreement can be renegotiated?
- How does the payer define medical necessity?
- Do co-payments apply to audiology claims? If so, what codes are they associated with?
- How will facilities and providers be notified of substantive changes to the agreement?
- Can the payer amend the contract without an authorized signature?
- Does the payer recognize CAQH credentialing?
- Are there any requirements for the practice to have a standard fee schedule/charge master?
- What are the timely claims filing requirements for the plan?
- What constitutes a "clean claim" for this payer?
- Can paper claims be submitted to this payer?
- Does the plan have any specific clinic hours or accessibility requirements?
- What are the plans' medical record retention requirements? Do they exceed state or Health Insurance Portability and Accountability Act (HIPAA) requirements?

- Does the fee schedule address all of the items and services you provide to your general population of patients? What is allowable for each HCPCS and CPT® code? How are unlisted codes such as CPT® code 92700 (unlisted otorhinolargyngological item or service), L9900 (orthotic and prosthetic supply, accessory, and/or service component of another HCPCS), V5298 (hearing aid not otherwise classified), and V5299 (hearing service, miscellaneous) processed?
- Is the hearing aid benefit an inclusive benefit? In other words, does the total benefit amount include all items and services related to the evaluation, procurement, fitting, and adjustment of the hearing aid being dispensed or is the benefit paid on a fee for service, per code basis?
- Are the hearing aid allowable amounts in the fee schedule reimbursed as a percentage of billed charges? If so, what is the percentage?
- When billing hearing aids to the third-party payer, is it required that the manufacturer's invoice for the hearing aids be included with the claim? If yes, is the practice reimbursed merely for the fitting of the device and the invoice cost of the hearing aid only? Is the practice reimbursed for a percentage above the invoice cost?

It is important that each practice have a strong grasp of their own practice philosophy, financial needs, and operational limitations as they review each payer agreement and determine if the benefits of participation outweigh the costs of participation (Gesme, 2015). It is important that practices know how to calculate the breakeven point of their practice (A Guide to Itemizing Professional Services, 2012). This determines the minimum amount they can accept for each given item and service. Many third-party fee schedules are based on some calculation, typically a fixed percentage, and often from a given year of the Medicare Prospective Fee Schedule.

Practices need to be willing to negotiate with payers to create a written agreement that is a "win-

win" for all parties involved. Providers need to make realistic requests consistent with other payers and state and federal insurance laws. Also, again, practices need to determine what the pros and cons of participation are with each payer. If providers are ever unsure of some of the contract terms, they should consider hiring an insurance consultant and/or an attorney who specializes in health care and/or contract law to assist them. Audiologists should always attempt to negotiate for what they require from the agreement (Jones, 2006). Contracting communications with the payer should occur in writing whenever possible. It is also important to not sign the agreement until all of the questions have been addressed. It is possible that it can be more advantageous to not sign the agreement and be an out-of-network provider for the plan.

Credentialing

Contracting typically precedes credentialing; the process of credentialing is when the facility and provider collect data and each of the provider's professional education and qualifications are verified, and typically begins after the facility has decided to proceed with their enrollment in a specific third-party payer arrangement. These qualifications include, but are not limited to:

- Relevant academic and clinical background and training
- State licensure
- NPI
- Liability insurance (Aetna, 2015)

The third-party payer determines the rules surrounding who can and cannot be credentialed providers within their network. In many situations, hearing aid dispensers, audiology assistants, and/or technicians are prohibited from being credentialed providers in health insurance plans. It is important to ask credentialing questions as part of your contract review process. Providers need to complete their credentialing process before they can see members of an insurance plan as an in-network provider; the completion of the contracting and credentialing process delineates an in-network provider from an out-of-network provider.

Contract Renewals

The vast majority of third-party payer agreements automatically renew ("evergreen") each year on the anniversary of the eligibility date (Mosby, 2009). It is important for each practice to review (if available on the payer website), or request in writing, a copy of their current payer fee schedules for each insurance product (i.e., PPO, POS, HMO, Medicare Part C) they are contracted to provide. It is also important that practices are aware of how they are to be informed of substantive changes to the third-party agreement and what their rights and responsibilities are when changes are made. This information is typically addressed in the initial agreement itself or in the clarification period of contract negotiations.

Contract Renegotiation

Contract renegotiation typically follows the same course as that of initial contracting with the only difference being the practice needs to determine the time frame and steps required to request a renegotiation of their third-party payer agreement. This process can vary payer to payer.

If the practice has not maintained a copy of their original third-party payer agreement, it is recommended that they review the guidance available on the payer website for their state and request a copy of the payer's current provider agreement. It is also vital that the practice have a current copy of the payer fee schedule for every insurance product that they are contracted with prior to beginning the renegotiation process. Providers must proceed with contract renegotiations knowing what they want and why they deserve it based on solid data and evidence, with a willingness to terminate the agreement if their basic terms are not met. Practices lose all leverage in a negotiation process if they are ill prepared and, ultimately, unwilling to terminate the agreement. It is important that

these renegotiation actions and processes occur in writing as much as possible. Unwritten terms and agreements tend to be problematic, especially if they conflict with existing written aspects of the agreement (i.e., negotiations related to hearing aid upgrades) or they affect claims processing (i.e., fee schedule changes).

Conclusion

Managed care has always been commonplace in an audiology practice. It is the growth of third-party coverage of hearing aids that has made the stakes much higher and the need to understand third-party payers, contracting, and credentialing more important. Every practice should have an individual who is responsible for having copies of the third-party agreements and fee schedules, as well as a working knowledge of the requirements, guidelines, and contractual obligations of each agreement. Audiologists are voluntary participants in managed care. If they choose to participate, they need to do so with an understanding of their rights and responsibilities before they proceed.

References

Accountable Care Organizations (ACO). (2015, January 6). Retrieved October 15, 2015 from https://www.cms.gov/Medicare/Medicare-Fee-for-Service-Payment/ACO/index.html?redirect=%2Faco.

A Guide to Itemizing Your Professional Services. (2012). American Academy of Audiology. Retrieved October 16, 2015 from http://www.audiology.org/sites/default/files/20141001_AAA_Guide2ItemizingUrProfeServices.pdf.

Carve-out. (n.d.). *Mosby's Medical Dictionary*, 8th edition. (2009). Retrieved October 16, 2015 from http://medical-dictionary.thefreedictionary.com/carve-out.

Clean Claim. (n.d.). *Medical Dictionary for the Health Professions and Nursing*. (2012). Retrieved October 19, 2015 from http://medical-dictionary.thefreedictionary.com/clean+claim.

CAQH. (n.d.). Retrieved October 19, 2015 from http://www.caqh.org/.

Evergreen Contract. (n.d.) *Mosby's Medical Dictionary*, 8th edition. (2009). Retrieved October 19, 2015 from http://medical-dictionary.thefreedictionary.com/evergreen+contract.

Gesme, D. H. & Wiseman, M. (n.d.). How to negotiate with health care plans. Retrieved October 19, 2015 from http://www.ncbi.nlm.nih.gov/pmc/articles/PMC2900878/.

Health Care Professionals: Joining the Network FAQs. (n.d.). Retrieved October 19, 2015 from https://www.aetna.com/faqs-health-insurance/health-care-professionals-join-network.html.

Health Maintenance Organization (HMO) Definition. (2010, September 17). Retrieved October 15, 2015 from https://www.healthinsurance.org/glossary/health-maintenance-organizations-hmos/.

Hearing Aid Insurance Mandates: Ensuring Access to Sound One State at a Time. (n.d.). Retrieved October 15, 2015 from http://www.agbell.org/Document.aspx?id=1805.

Incident to Services. (2015, November 24). Retrieved April 1, 2016 from https://med.noridianmedicare.com/web/jeb/topics/incident-to-services.

Jones, C. (2006, November/December). Negotiating a contract with a health plan. Retrieved October 19, 2015 from http://www.aafp.org/fpm/2006/1100/p49.html.

Medicaid Definition | Investopedia. (2005, March 03). Retrieved October 15, 2015 from http://www.investopedia.com/terms/m/medicaid.asp.

Point-of-Service Plan (POS). (n.d.). Retrieved October 15, 2015 from http://healthcoverageguide.org/reference-guide/coverage-types/point-of-service-plan-pos/.

The Lexicon of Supervision: CMS Versus ACGME Defined Terms. (2011, July 5). Retrieved October 16, 2015 from http://www.hallrender.com/library/articles/862/070511HLN.html.

Third-party Reimbursement. (n.d.) *Mosby's Medical Dictionary*, 8th edition. (2009). Retrieved October 15 2015 from http://medical-dictionary.thefreedictionary.com/third-party+reimbursement.

What Is Medicare? (n.d.). Retrieved October 15, 2015 from www.medicare.gov/...medicare/...medicare/what-is-medicare.html.

CHAPTER 5

Itemizing Professional Services for Hearing Aids

Stephanie Sjoblad

Introduction

When one reviews the headlines in hearing health-care news or receives updates from national advisory panels regarding hearing care there is a common theme. There is a growing interest in making hearing care more accessible and more affordable as there is a concern that few adults with hearing loss are using hearing aids. In October 2015, the President's Council of Advisors on Science and Technology (PCAST) issued a report on Aging America & Hearing Loss: Imperative of Improved Hearing Technologies with recommendations designed to improve access to hearing care for adults. The PCAST report outlines a number of barriers related to the low uptake of hearing aids today with a strong emphasis on the high cost. At the same time, there appears to be no shortage of companies trying to capitalize on the 37.5 million Americans with hearing loss (Blackwell, Lucas, & Clarke 2014). Over the past decade, hearing aid dispensing practices have been popping up in drug stores, Costco is gaining market share, and insurance companies are setting up marketing channels to get hearing aids directly into the hands of the patient. It would seem hearing aids and hearing health care has become commoditized.

Most audiologists enter the profession with a desire to help people improve their quality of life. Many have no prior background in business or have an understanding of billing and coding for their services. The bundled billing model was the norm for over 30 years, so most audiologists have not given much thought to placing value on their services; the emphasis was on dispensing hearing aids. This chapter will empower the audiologist who is looking to remain competitive in changing times. The reader will discover the process that the UNC Hearing and Communication Center underwent at their community-based clinic to move to an itemized billing model, as well as read some success stories from other practices that have moved to itemization.

Unbundling versus Itemizing

When the UNC-HCC clinic started the process of placing value on professional services, the buzz word often associated with this process was "unbundling." To unbundle is to separate (dictionary.com, 2015). To itemize is to break down (a whole) into its constituent parts (dictionary.com, 2015). The nomenclature that will be used through the remainder of this chapter will be "itemize."

Background

In August 2002, the University of North Carolina at Chapel Hill welcomed the first cohort of students to complete their AuD degree. The arrival of these students was a turning point for the program in thinking about how to value time with patients. At the time, the university had a small, on-campus hearing aid dispensing practice, sufficient for teaching three to five students the ins and outs of hearing aid fitting and follow-up. The patients paid for the device at the conclusion of an often very long trial period and were charged a very, very small fee that was considered the "fitting fee." They began to think more seriously about the message this was sending to consumers, as well as the message that was being sent to the students who were now training to become doctors of audiology.

Around this same time, there was some beginning discussion within the profession about the practice of unbundling or itemizing for the device in addition to professional services. The literature on the topic of itemizing dates back more than 15 years when Toni Gitles discussed the consumer's view of the audiologist as one of a sales or service person, not a professional (Gitles, 1999). Today, there are more hearing aid distribution channels than ever before. A Google search for the word "hearing aids" produced over 27 million options in less than one second. When perusing these online options, there is a very clear theme. Many of these channels suggest to consumers that the professional expertise of the audiologist is unnecessary. In collaboration with the American Academy of Audiolgy (AAA), the UNC-Hearing and Communication Center (UNC-HCC) developed the Hearing Aid Billing Practices Survey which was distributed to the entire membership in early 2011 and also in 2012. The survey provided some great insight into the concerns members of AAA had about itemizing. The most recent AAA Billing Practices Survey in 2012 revealed that 67% of practices remain bundled. This decades-old method of billing in audiology has certainly not helped to separate the importance of the professional from the limitations of the device.

As the team at the UNC-HCC clinic began to contemplate how they might change this, additional articles appeared. In 2003, Dennis Van Vliet, stated "bundled pricing does not offer a full accounting of the clear scope of our services" (Van Vliet, 2003). In 2005, the UNC-HCC clinic was inspired by Patricia Gans' partially itemized model. This unique model included services for the duration of the "trial period" and then fee for service

henceforth (Nemes, 2004). In this model, the patient pays upfront professional fees which include quality assurance, the initial fitting, and two to three follow-up visits within the first 45 days. At that time, the UNC-HCC clinic had concerns a completely unbundled model may lead to less than optimal fitting should a patient forego certain procedures or visits in an effort to save money. Therefore, they established which key services are non-negotiable (i.e., electroacoustic analysis, probemic measures, etc.). Over the past 10 years, the concept of itemizing has continued to gain traction. In 2009, Robert Sweetow led an AAA Task Force to look at current hearing aid delivery models. Featured in *Audiology Today*, the two-part article discussed the advantages of itemizing and the ability to use a fair and unbundled-only schedule to promote our professional and specialized services. The Task Force also suggested a change in billing methods could promote increased reimbursement and help distinguish audiologists from non-audiologists who dispense. Finally, the Task Force emphasized very strongly that audiologists should never give away professional services for the purpose of selling a product (Sweetow, 2009b).

In theory, this is all well and good, but when the UNC-HCC clinic started on this journey, there was no evidence to support the concept that itemized billing would work. In 2004, the university training clinic was forced to move to a community-based location and there was more pressure to grow the business and ensure that the clinic was covering all costs. One year after opening the doors, the UNC-HCC clinic moved to an itemized billing model which now has more than a 10-year history of successful unbundled billing (Sjoblad-Warren, 2011).

Disclaimer

It is important to emphasize that the UNC-HCC clinic is a non-profit clinic and although a university training clinic for doctoral students of audiology, it is self-supported and self-sustaining. The UNC-HCC clinic is community-based and as such, receives no state funding. Thus, it functions essentially like a private practice clinic. The UNC-HCC clinic has its own budget, and must pay rent, salaries, overhead, and so on from clinical revenues much like any practice, facing the same economic challenges as those in the private sector. Additionally, due to continuous state budget cuts, the university training program is becoming more reliant on revenue generated by clinical services to help offset academic program expenses.

Considerations

Prior to moving to an itemized billing model in 2005, the UNC-HCC clinic often had days when 10 to 15 patients were seen, resulting in no revenue. In addition, an increasing number of patients presented to the clinic for a second opinion, having purchased hearing aids elsewhere. The clinic knew it needed to charge for its time, but did not know what that time was worth. Another consideration that was an enormous hurdle for the team was acknowledging that all time was valuable and not to be reluctant to charge for services. Other professionals charge for their expertise, from plumbers and hairstylists to physicians and attorneys. The UNC-HCC clinic began to contemplate, "Is there a better way to bill for services that will assign value to what we do as audiologists?" The UNC-HCC clinic spent several years finding its way and as a result this chapter can serve as a how-to guide for others who wish to follow the same path, albeit more quickly.

Calculating the Hourly Rate and Assigning Fees on the Superbill

The first step in moving to an itemized billing model is to complete a breakeven analysis and determine the minimal hourly rate that one must charge to keep the doors open. Unfortunately, the UNC-HCC clinic did not start with this method, but this chapter allows you to benefit from their experiences and do it correctly from the start. One cannot set up an appropriate fee schedule until one has established what it costs to run the business. Once the hourly rate is determined, one should create a superbill, utilizing proper codes for everything related to hearing aid delivery and au-

Breakeven Hourly Rate

Determine how many hours (annually) you can bill for services provided

Patient contact hours per week:	30 hours
Number of weeks worked per year:	48 weeks
Number of providers:	2 providers

30 x 48 x 2 = 2880

Figure 5–1. Calculating the breakeven hourly rate Part 1.

diologic rehabilitation. Audiologists can use both CPT® (Current Procedural Terminology) codes and HCPCS (Health Care Current Procedure Coding System) codes when establishing a fee schedule. Throughout this book and chapter you will find some of the current most relevant codes for hearing aid services.

According to the 2012 AAA Hearing Aid Billing Practices Survey, less than half (49%) of audiologists surveyed have calculated break-even analysis to determine what it costs to run their practice, stating they were either arbitrarily choosing rates or using the going rate in the area or some other method. With or without a degree in business, it is fairly simple to calculate the cost of doing business (Foltner, 2009).

1. Establish annual contact hours:
   - Determine how many hours per week one can see/bill patients. Although the practice may operate 40 hours per week, one must consider the time that is related to direct patient contact.
   - Calculate the number of weeks per year that one actually sees patients (factor in vacation, holidays, sick days, and professional leave).
   - Determine the number of providers in the practice.
   - Multiply the hours per week by weeks per year by the number of providers (Figure 5–1).

2. Calculate the operating costs for the practice. Ideally this would be broken down into several different expense categories, including:
   - Personnel (salary/benefits)
   - Clinic expenses (rent, utilities, phone, advertising, etc.)
   - Cost of goods (all things you buy for resale)
3. Determine the break-even hourly rate.
   - Subtract the cost of goods from total annual clinic expenses, and divide the remaining amount by the "annual contact hours" established in Step 1.
   - This is the break-even hourly rate (Figure 5–2).
4. Add in desired profit.
   - Take annual expenses less cost of goods, add desired profit, and divide this number by the annual contact hours.
   - This is the hourly rate including the desired profit (Figure 5–3).

In the above-itemized model, the cost of goods has been excluded from the equation, as it is expected one will collect, at a minimum, dollar for dollar on the cost of products. In most clinics, there will still be some markup over the invoice cost to cover situations when one cannot collect the hourly rate. For example, the current reimbursement from Medicare for a comprehensive hearing evaluation rarely would cover the cost of doing business in the time one takes to complete that patient visit.

Once determining the hourly rate, the next step is to apply this rate to the various services offered in the clinic based on the amount of time it

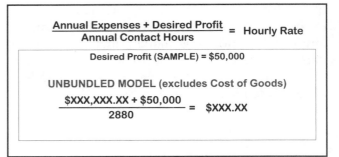

Figure 5–3. Hourly rate and desired profit calculation Part 3.

typically takes to perform this task. For example, if the hourly rate is determined to be $100.00 per hour, this would be the equivalent of $25.00 per 15-minute intervals. If you see a patient for 15 minutes to perform a hearing aid check, you would want to be sure you are billing at least $25.00 for that 15-minute appointment.

Considerations

In-network insurance coverage: If your clinic is "in-network" for hearing aid services, start by getting a fee schedule from all current "in-network" insurance plans to determine the maximum amount the insurance company will pay for any given service. While it's important to keep the hourly rate in mind, one should be sure to set the rate for any service at or above the maximum amount covered by insurance. For example, if a hearing aid service (V5020–Conformity Evaluation) is covered by ABC insurance company for $75.00, one would want to be sure at a minimum they are billing all patients $75.00 for V5020; otherwise, money will be left on the table. This could be considered your usual and customary fee.

Hearing Aid Pricing

As one works to determine the price for hearing aids for the clinic, one must realize that the invoice cost for the hearing aid is not the actual cost to the practice. There are other direct and indirect

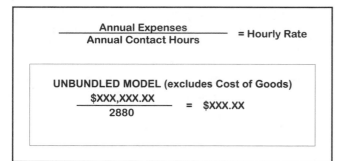

Figure 5–2. Hourly rate calculation Part 2.

product costs that may need to be recouped with a mark-up on the device. A practice with a high percentage of Medicare patients in their payer mix may require a larger margin when setting hearing aid prices than a practice that sees patients predominantly under the age of 65. It cannot be overly stressed that each clinic or practice must set their own rates as the rate is entirely dependent on covering expenses for your clinic.

Frequency of Evaluating Fees

Annually, the clinic should re-establish their break-even rate and then re-establish how much money it will take per hour to simply keep the doors open. The process of establishing fees is not a one-time event, but one that should be re-evaluated at a minimum of once per year as expenses and cost of goods change. This will ensure the fees for services one provides cover the current annual operation costs, a valuable exercise that will enable the practice to prosper year in and year out.

Evidence-Based Practice

While the process for the UNC-HCC clinic to move to an itemized model took place over a long period of time, throughout the process the team was committed to always looking to the evidence and ensuring that they were using best practices when working with patients. When fitting hearing aids, one should look to the Guidelines for the Audiologic Management of Adult Hearing Impairment established by the American Academy of Audiology (AAA, 2006). The audiologists at the UNC-HCC clinic find that when patients are informed of best practices and evidence-based measures, they are agreeable to undergo the necessary procedures and return for the follow-up visits. It is also logical to charge patients for all visits because they can see the benefit of your services when utilizing evidence-based practice. The UNC-HCC clinic billing model separates the fee for services from the device, establishes value for the professional expertise of the audiologist, and sets the stage for a successful fitting. The UNC-HCC clinic believes

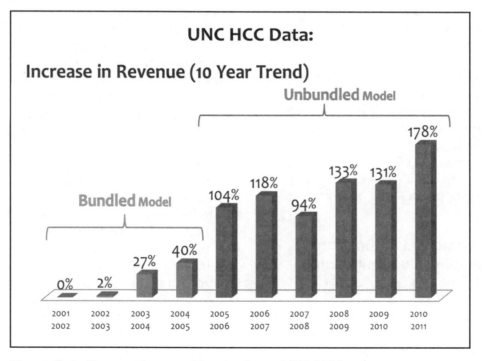

Figure 5–4. Ten-year impact of itemization at UNC-HCC.

there is a strong connection between the introduction of more testing, expanded protocols and validation tools, and success of their itemized business model. A graph showing revenue generated from hearing aids *and* professional services over a 10-year period shows that itemizing has been favorable for the health of the UNC-HCC clinic (Figure 5–4).

UNC-HCC Clinic Model of Care

Step One: Hearing Evaluation

When patients call the clinic to schedule a hearing evaluation, the front office team will gather all pertinent demographic and insurance information and schedule the patient. The appointment for a hearing evaluation is typically a 1-hour visit, though sometimes it may be 1.5 hours. The audiologist will conduct a thorough case history, complete diagnostic testing, review test results, and discuss recommendations with the patient. The patient will be given an overview of the process utilized at the UNC-HCC clinic if the patient is a candidate for treatment (hearing aids, assistive technology, communication strategies, etc.) and it will be determined if they are interested in proceeding. The patient will check out and schedule a follow-up visit for the Hearing Aid Evaluation appointment if they wish to pursue treatment. The audiologist will send a comprehensive report to the patient's referring physician or provider including all findings and recommendations. If the patient is self-referred, permission is obtained to send a comprehensive report to their Primary Care Physician (PCP) as well. The clinic believes a partnership with the PCP is in the patient's best interest.

Step Two: Hearing Aid Evaluation– aka The Functional Communication Assessment

The Hearing Aid Evaluation (HAE) appointment has established CPT® codes, a HCPCS code, and an S code that may be utilized. Check with your fee schedules for the best choice. Medicare does not recognize any of these codes as a covered service.

CPT® codes:
- 92590 (Hearing aid examination and selection, monaural)
  - 92591 (Binaural)

HCPCS code:
- V5010 Assessment for hearing

S code:
- S0618 Audiometry for an HAE to determine the level and degree of hearing loss

Over the years, there was much discussion about charging for this appointment among the audiology team at the UNC-HCC clinic. Some of the more senior clinicians were accustomed to "bundling" the HAE into the hearing aid price and were reluctant to ask the patient to pay separately for this appointment. However, if the patient does not purchase hearing aids at the conclusion of the HAE appointment, then they have been given an hour of services for free. An argument in favor of charging for this service was "how could we, as a training clinic, suggest to our students that they are becoming Doctors of Audiology to give away their services?"

In 2008, this discussion ended as the Hearing Aid Evaluation appointment was renamed more appropriately a Functional Communication Assessment (FCA). The UNC-HCC clinic FCA appointment now included both objective and subjective methods for developing a treatment plan for the patient (Sweetow, 2007) and the emphasis was taken from the ears and began looking at the whole person. The FCA appointment begins with a pre-fitting assessment tool, such as the Characteristics of Amplification Tool (COAT), the Abbreviate Profile of Hearing Aid Benefit (APHAB), or the Expected Consequences of Hearing Aid Ownership (ECHO). The use of these assessment tools enables the audiologist to gather subjective information from the patient about their motivation, their concerns about benefit, cost, cosmetics, and so on prior to the appointment. It also allows the patient to reflect on their personal reasons to improve their hearing.

Loudness Discomfort Levels

The UNC-HCC clinic formally used to measure Loudness Discomfort Levels (LDLs) during the Hearing Evaluation appointment, but transitioned this test to be a part of the patient's FCA.

Speech in Noise Testing and Other Objective Tests

To obtain a better understanding of how patients process sound in background noise, speech in noise testing is completed. The UNC-HCC clinic utilizes the QuickSIN test. Additionally, the audiologist may elect to conduct other tests such as the TEN (HL) to assess cochlear dead regions, and the Acceptable Noise Level (ANL), the Performance Perceptual Test (PPT), and so on.

Lifestyle Assessment

After gathering additional objective data about how the patient processes sound in more complex environments and loudness tolerances, the consultation continues utilizing a Lifestyle Assessment form developed by the UNC-HCC clinic. The Lifestyle Assessment form enables the audiologist to interview the patient to learn more about patient considerations, such as home and work environments, challenging listening environments, phone needs, vision and dexterity issues, and so on. After learning more about the client's personal lifestyle and communication needs, the audiologist and patient work together to determine three communication situations the patient hopes to improve by the end of the treatment process. The UNC-HCC clinic utilizes a modified version of the Client Oriented Scale of Improvement (COSI) and works to establish the patient's present ability, desired ability, and realistic ability in each of their given listening situations. This provides a way to re-examine the most important issues to the patient at each follow-up visit and allows a way to measure outcomes at the conclusion of the fitting/adjustment process. The FCA appointment duration can be up to 1.5 hours in length, but provides a more comprehensive picture of the patient's hearing and communication

needs. At the conclusion of this appointment the audiologist will make recommendations to the patient for technology (hearing aids, connectivity devices, FM) as well as audiologic rehabilitation such as communication strategies training, auditory training, Better Hearing Workshop classes, and so on. Working with the patient, the audiologist will help them choose the devices and tools that best meet their needs and budget. If custom ear molds are required, the audiologist would take ear impressions at this appointment.

The UNC-HCC clinic was already charging patients for this service, but adoption of the FCA demonstrates a methodical and comprehensive approach to the selection of the hearing instruments and the development of a treatment plan beyond amplification. The advantage of this process is to emphasize the audiologist's knowledge and skills in assisting the development of a treatment plan. The emphasis is taken from the "device" and the focus is now on the total treatment plan.

If the patient has insurance coverage for CPT® codes 92590 or 92591, one would bill the patient or the third-party payer at the conclusion of the visit, regardless of whether the patient purchased hearing aids. The audiologist would also charge for each ear mold impression (V5275) and each ear mold (V5264) at the HAE/FCA appointment. This helps ensure that if the patient elected to cancel the hearing aid order upon leaving the clinic, the fees for the service of taking the impressions and the non-refundable ear molds would already have been collected.

Step Three: Hearing Aid Fitting Process

Hearing Aid Check

The following CPT® codes are utilized for visual and listening checks:

- 92592 Hearing aid check; monaural
- 92593 Hearing aid check; binaural

When the hearing aid(s)/earmold(s) arrive from the manufacturers, the first step is to perform an inspection to ensure the clinic received what was ordered. The person checking in the devices (often a graduate assistant and could be an audiologist's assistant) would match the color, style, materials, and so on with the order form and the patient's chart note and complete a listening check.

Electro-Acoustic Analysis (EAA)

There are two CPT® codes for performing an electroacoustic evaluation:

- 92594 Electroacoustic evaluation for hearing aid; monaural
- 92595 Electroacoustic evaluation for hearing aid; binaural

Next, every hearing aid received from the manufacturer must undergo and pass electroacoustic analysis (EAA) prior to the patient's fitting appointment. The importance of this step is well documented in the AAA Task Force Guidelines for Treatment of Adult Hearing Impairment (AAA, 2006). But taking it a step further, if one is going to charge a fee for service, for every visit, one must be confident that the devices are working properly before the patient leaves the office. In 2009, the UNC-HCC clinic completed a retrospective study to assess what percentage of new hearing aid orders passed ANSI standards/EAA on arrival from the manufacturer. Twelve percent of brand new orders failed inspection; eighteen percent of repaired hearing aids failed inspection. Completing an EAA is the only way to guarantee the device is working to specifications when it is delivered to the patient. At the UNC-HCC clinic, it is rare that a patient returns shortly after the fitting with an ill-functioning hearing aid because it was not working or not truly fixed after a manufacturer repair. There are CPT® codes for this procedure and therefore it is important to bill these codes to establish the value of the service, both with the patient and with third-party payers.

Hearing Aid Fitting

There are Healthcare Common Procedural Coding System (HCPCS) codes for services one should provide during the fitting process:

- V5020 – Conformity evaluation (may include real ear measures, validation, functional gain measures)
- V5014 – Repair/modification of a hearing aid
- V5011 – Fitting/orientation/checking of hearing aid

On the day of the fitting, the patient's hearing test results and LDLs are uploaded into the verification system prior to bringing the patient into the fitting office for their appointment. The process of transferring data from the audiometer to computer to verification system and back has greatly improved over the years and can now be transferred in a matter of moments. The patient is seated in the chair in front of the verification system. They are shown their new devices. The audiologist will inspect the ear canal, insert the hearing aids to check fit/comfort, then remove the device to set up for real ear probe microphone measures (REM).

The audiologist explains to the patient that the REM procedure will take their hearing range and their ear canal resonance into consideration and enable customization of the fitting using researched-based prescriptive targets. The audiologist will set the manufacturer's software at the maximum adaptation or experience level when running initial REM curves. They will run three curves before making any changes in the fitting software (soft speech, average speech, and MPO). Then, the audiologist will make software adjustments and remeasure until targets are met throughout the speech range and have maximized the patient's Speech Intelligibility Index and the patient's audibility. REM is an evidence-based procedure that enables the audiologist to demonstrate their knowledge and skill and establish their value. Most audiologists who do not use REM would be very surprised to see how often first fit does not provide appropriate audibility for the patient. Additionally, when one fails to use REM, they have not demonstrated to their patient a distinctive service that could not be performed by a technician entering the audiometric data and selecting first fit. As a billable code, REM may become a leading source of revenue for clinics as market distribution channels expand and patients opt to purchase hearing aids from other sources. Clinics that can demonstrate their knowledge and expertise by using REM and other evidence-based procedures when selecting and programming hearing aids will be a step ahead in the coming days.

Orientation and Adjustments

After matching prescriptive targets with REM, the audiologist will assess the patient's preferences for sound and adjust the volume as needed, utilizing the manufacturer's adaptation levels. Patients are informed the goal is to be at 100% of targets to maximize their audibility and speech intelligibility. However, if a patient has had long duration of hearing loss without amplification this cannot always be achieved the day of the initial fitting. Prior to saving and disconnecting the patient from the computer, the audiologist may add a phone and/or t-coil program. The audiologist considers any other necessary adjustments needed in helping the patient meet their COSI goals.

Counseling and Orientation

The UNC-HCC clinic usually devotes 1 hour for the initial hearing aid fitting and counseling appointment. The first 15 to 20 minutes are spent programming with REM, with the remainder of the appointment reviewing the care and use of the hearing aids and discussing communication strategies. Prior to the patient leaving the fitting room, the audiologist will review the terms of purchase and paperwork with the patient.

Purchase Agreement

The purchase agreement the UNC-HCC clinic developed has necessary information as required by North Carolina state law. It will be important to ensure one checks their licensing laws as one develops their purchase agreement as these vary from state to state. The UNC-HCC clinic utilizes both a purchase agreement and an invoice. The first item on the purchase agreement is the fee for professional services, stating that the professional ser-

vice fees are non-refundable (varies by state law). Additionally, the purchase agreement has the device price (by device), as well as the warranty terms and information about policies. The UNC-HCC clinic refrains from using the terminology "trial period" in discussions and on the purchase agreement. Instead, the preferred term is "evaluation and adjustment period." The audiologist will review the purchase agreement with the patient and discuss all the terms. The patient checks out at the front desk with their signed purchase agreement and the superbill with all the appropriate codes circled for services rendered to prepare the devices for the appointment as well as all services completed during the appointment with the patient.

Payment

All monetary transactions occur at the front desk with the practice manager. The audiology team is discouraged from walking the patient to the checkout desk. The codes from the superbill are entered into the accounting system and an invoice is generated for the patient. The patient pays the entire invoice by check or credit card prior to leaving the clinic. The invoice has a detailed itemization of each professional service that was rendered and the corresponding CPT® and/or HCPCS codes. The invoice also has a separate line item for the hearing devices, so the devices and services are itemized. If the patient has an insurance benefit and is "in-network," collect whatever is the allowable patient responsibility at the time of the fitting and then process the claim. Either way, the patient leaves with documentation of all the services that were provided during their visit. Follow up appointments are scheduled at the time of check out.

Step Four: Follow-Up Care/ Audiologic Rehabilitation

The UNC-HCC clinic policy includes 45 days of services in the upfront fees paid by the patient for most purchases. This "partially unbundled" service model for the fitting was the decision that was made to ensure the patient will come back for necessary follow-up appointments until the evaluation and adjustment period is over. At each of these follow-up visits, the audiologist will circle the superbill with whatever procedures may have been performed during the appointment. For example, if at the subsequent appointment, the audiologist had modified an earmold for discomfort and counseled on how to insert the devices, then they would circle the corresponding services on the superbill. The UNC-HCC clinic set up a code to alert the front desk when a patient is still in their 45-day evaluation period. When the patient checks out, they receive another invoice with a detailed list of each service that was provided, but the invoice would indicate the fee was pre-paid. This system reinforces to the patient each time they visit the clinic what services were performed and that the services were pre-paid, not free.

Final Fitting Follow-Up Appointment

At the final fitting follow-up appointment, the audiologist will go through a clinic checklist that helps with training students, but also allows one to be sure the patient is a confident and satisfied user before discharging them to longer-term follow-up. The checklist covers items such as insertion and removal capability, device comfort, device cleaning, use of devices/changing programs, and the use of any connectivity/accessories. The audiologist will review the patient's satisfaction with the services at the UNC-HCC clinic and revisit the patient's original COSI communication goals. It is very rewarding to have the patients rank their "after treatment" goals and discover how that differs from pre-treatment. Most patients at the UNC-HCC clinic report dramatic improvement at the conclusion of the treatment process. In the rare instances where the patient is not meeting their expected performance, the audiologist will recommend continued audiologic rehabilitation which may be the Better Hearing Workshop classes, additional accessories, auditory training, and/or more counseling. The UNC-HCC clinic encourages all patients to attend the Better Hearing Workshops,

especially encouraging those who need more hand-holding. Over the past 14 years, the clinic return for credit rate has been less than 1% to 2% annually, well below national averages. The process outlined in this chapter, which has been used by the UNC-HCC clinic for over 10 years, creates successful outcomes essentially every time.

The last thing the audiologist will discuss with the patient before they graduate from their "evaluation and adjustment period" is the clinic fee policies for future appointments. In efforts to keep hearing care costs as low as possible, the UNC-HCC clinic favors the "pay as you go model," though an optional service plan program was added in July 2013. To date, only two people have elected to purchase the service plan.

Step Five: Maintenance

Several years ago, the UNC-HCC clinic changed its policy for hearing aid check-ups from "as needed" to scheduling regular check-ups for its patients. In most instances, patients will benefit from a minimum of two recheck appointments per year, at 6-month intervals. Each clinician uses their own discretion if a patient needs care more frequently. At this appointment, the audiologist would review the patient's case history to be sure there have not been any changes in hearing or other symptoms and discuss triumphs and/or disappointments. The visit includes an otoscopic inspection and discussion of findings with the patient. Occasionally, cerumen management may be needed and patients pay for this service if needed. The hearing aids are serviced with small parts replacement, such as tubing, filters, wax traps, mic covers, and so on. The devices are placed in a drying system and a listening check is completed. The audiologist may verify patient usage with the device's data logging software, review experience level, and make programming adjustments as needed. If the device fails the listening check, the audiologist may replace receivers as needed and/or conduct electroacoustic analyses. Patients check out with a superbill that has all the provided services circled. At the annual visit, the audiologist will repeat the following and recommend an updated EAA as needed. Even though the patient is "in warranty" with the manufacturer, they pay for the services the audiologist provided in the office. This has all been very clearly explained on the purchase agreement and most patients understand this policy. If it is problematic to "pay as they go," the patient is reminded of the goal of keeping upfront costs as low as possible and it is suggested that the patient may wish to purchase a service plan if that would give them peace of mind.

Service Plans

The UNC-HCC clinic has favored the "'pay as you go'" model, but there is certainly a place for service plans for some patients. The UNC-HCC clinic has chosen to outline the service plan option at the conclusion of the "evaluation and adjustment period." Another business model would be to outline on the purchase order that service is covered for a certain time period, what it covers, and what the cost is for needed services. It is important in this new climate of hearing care that patients are comparing apples to apples. If a clinic suggests that Brand A hearing aids cost $5,000/pair but doesn't detail the breakdown for the patient of the cost of fitting, service, and devices, the patient will be comparing apples to oranges if they find the same Brand A hearing aids online or retail for a fraction of that cost. A practice does not necessarily have to unbundle to demonstrate value. Itemization of product and services will also demonstrate value and enable a more appropriate comparison for the price shopper.

Transitioning to Itemized Billing at End of Warranty

Early in the process of the UNC-HCC clinic's move to itemize billing, the team began to stop giving away services once the manufacturer's warranty period had concluded. Interestingly, it was at the conclusion of a visit with a patient who was a retired dentist that prompted a different viewpoint. This patient, a retired faculty dentist, was outside

of his "warranty period" and he stressed the importance of recognizing the value of services provided and stated one should not hesitate to charge patients for their time and expertise. Changing the purchase agreement to clearly reflect fee for service once the warranty expires can be a good segue for clinics that are currently bundled to move to itemization.

Caring for Patients Who Purchased Elsewhere

We all receive inquiries from patients who have purchased devices elsewhere, either moving away from their original provider or wanting another opinion. In the future, we may see more patients coming to us for our services only, not the device, and consequently, we will not benefit from any mark-up on product. This is less concerning if the clinic is billing its hourly rate for each patient visit. Every patient that comes to the UNC-HCC clinic for service is treated the same regardless of where they purchased their devices. The audiologist will attempt to help the patient solve the problem that brought them to the clinic; sometimes it is just a good cleaning of their devices. Often, the case history and otoscopic inspection reveal a new hearing evaluation is needed and other times the patient needs their hearing aids reprogrammed. The UNC-HCC clinic has programming software for most major manufacturers. In the instance where the patient has a device that is "locked" or proprietary, one may be limited in how one can help them. It may be that after a good cleaning, all one can do is demonstrate to the patient how much of the speech range is audible using REM. Many patients elect to pay for REM, which then gives them the ability to make more informed decisions. Perhaps after the visit, they will go back to their original provider (if they can) for adjustments. More often, patients elect to move forward with newer technology at the UNC-HCC clinic because the audiologist has demonstrated their expertise. As more patients begin to purchase "starter" devices or less expensive devices elsewhere, there is always an opportunity to showcase our skills as audiologists if they visit us for our opinion.

Historical Information

The UNC-HCC clinic has been partially unbundled and has itemized since 2005. Over the past 10 years, tweaking the billing structure and improving consistency in billing practices among providers continues. The superbill is updated to improve the utilization of proper coding between providers for the same appointment type. Every patient, whether a walk-in patient or a scheduled patient, checks-out with a superbill "circled" indicating all services rendered. The UNC-HCC clinic's office manager generates an invoice for every single patient to take home that lists all the services provided and collects full payment the day the service is rendered for all out-of-network patients, and collects allowables if a patient is in-network and has a hearing aid benefit. Each time the patient is seen within the 45-day evaluation and adjustment period, they check out with an invoice that details all the services rendered, which depicts a zero dollar amount indicating these services were pre-paid in the professional fees at the time of the fitting. It is important for patients to see what services have been provided each time they see the audiologist.

Success Stories from their Clinics

Hearing Solutions of North Carolina, Salisbury, North Carolina

Lorin Oden, AuD, started itemizing because she was tired of patients only seeing the total cost for the "little piece of plastic" they were purchasing and frequently asking her "Why does this cost so much?" as they held up their hearing aids. She was frustrated the patient had no concept of the importance of her knowledge and expertise, nor the various services she provided to "make that hearing aid work." Dr. Oden worked at an ENT clinic for many years and when she first learned about itemized billing, suggested to the physicians they change the way they do business. The ENT practice hired an outside consultant to review the itemized business model she learned about from the UNC-HCC clinic and her idea was vetoed as not feasible. She also reported that ultimately the ENT physicians were not interested in change.

In March 2011, Dr. Oden opened a private practice clinic in Salisbury, North Carolina, and itemization was the chosen billing model from its inception. She is methodical in explaining to patients that her services are separate from the hearing aids and reports the patients "get it."

Hearing Solutions of North Carolina provides quarterly cleaning and hearing aid checks as part of their battery package, which patients pay for as part of their accessories package. Therefore, patients come in on a quarterly basis to pick up their batteries and have their devices cleaned at the same time. Patients pay for this service package up front, which means they are not charged additionally every time they come in for this particular service. The practice has set aside 1 hour each day which they call "open clinic" for walk-ins and checks. If the visit proves to be more complex than a "clean and check" an additional appointment is scheduled and the patient is charged for any services provided.

This has also provided consistency for those patients who receive their hearing aids through a third party or discount program. Hearing Solutions of North Carolina participates in several third-party payer and discount programs such as TruHearing, Hearing Care Solutions, as the fee they pay Dr. Oden for her professional services covers her hourly rate. However, once the adaption period is complete, patients then must pay out of pocket for their appointments. Dr. Oden will see these patients for a six-month and annual clean and check and the patient pays for all services rendered at each of those appointments. When Dr. Oden opened her practice, she developed a fee schedule and every service is a fee based on her hourly rate. She created a Hearing Rehabilitation Worksheet that assists her when talking to new patients. The worksheet lists all the necessary steps for a successful hearing aid fitting. Dr. Oden reviews all the components that go into a successful outcome and the associated fee for each service (diagnostic testing, ear impressions, earmolds, professional services, accessories, and the hearing aid) with the patient. Dr. Oden shared that the services and accessories fees are constant regardless of the technology level chosen. She stated it separates her from the hearing aid and she has no regrets in her decision to use an itemized billing model (Oden, 2016).

Audiology Experts, Arlington, Texas

Kristin Robbins, AuD, of Audiology Experts in Arlington, Texas, shared that itemization and service agreements have allowed her practice to provide patient care for a broader patient population in its geographic area. When the practice moved to itemization, it had the advantage of starting at the beginning of the calendar year. Dr. Robbins completed the crucial first steps of determining the cost of doing business per hour and reviewing what services she provided. Dr. Robbins had a fee for each service broken down. Initially the practice was bundled and presented these new options only to those who came from other practices. As her practice began to unbundle/itemize with each new patient, she would explain her service agreement option during the hearing aid evaluation and patients would choose their preferred service package at the end of their trial period.

Audiology Experts offers a no-charge consult to patients who have purchased elsewhere. This consultation is the time to review the patient's audiogram that is either brought with them or faxed from their former clinic. During this visit, they also evaluate the patient's dexterity, their ability to communicate, and the hearing aids are physically shown to the patient. The inspection of the hearing aids enables Dr. Robbins to obtain the hearing aid serial numbers. Armed with this information, the manufacturer is queried about the original purchase date and if there is any existing warranty information. Dr. Robbins will then assess whether the patient's present hearing aids are appropriate for their loss. If the devices are not appropriate, she will refrain from programming the hearing aids as they will never meet prescriptive targets. Instead, she will outline possible solutions, such as new earmolds, stronger receivers, or even replacement hearing aids to allow the patient to make an informed decision about the next steps.

While this practice offers this initial consult gratis, services it offers and the fees for cleaning, care, supplies, and so on are explained. If Dr. Robbins spends 30 minutes counseling the patient and/or their communication partner, cleaning the aids, or providing supplies, then the patient will be charged for the individual services/fees. When they have a patient whose hearing aids are appropriate for their hearing loss, the fees for service or the option of a service agreement are explained. The service agreement allows patients to pay up front for a year of service/programming and supplies, including the use of loaner hearing aids as needed. More than eighty-five percent of patients that "purchased elsewhere" sign up for the service plan, and more than ninety-five percent renew annually. The remaining five percent of patients convert to fee for service after a year or two of participating in the service plan.

Audiology Experts has seen itemization as an "administrative or business" strength, yet this model forced Dr. Robbins to evaluate her company each year in a different way. No longer was the question whether the practice was profitable from year to year, but where were the profit centers? She began to analyze if her business growth was a result of more patients with third-party insurance now coming to her practice to purchase. She was tracking patients that "purchased elsewhere" to assess whether they choose a service plan or preferred to pay fee for service. She also tracks long-term loyalty to see if new patients who formerly purchased elsewhere have remained with her clinic and eventually purchased new hearing aids from the practice. There was a learning curve but tracking data and being flexible to implement change have been vital to Dr. Robbins' success. The more she learned from mentors or from billing/coding trial and error in her own office or as changes occurred with insurance contracts, Dr. Robbins would institute changes or streamline services to be cost-effective. Dr. Robbins stressed that for this billing model to be successful, she has found there must be someone in the office dedicated to understanding the insurance contracts, administrative costs of running the office, and determining the prices of the services/service plan. It can be a daunting task to keep that information current and accurate. There can be challenges for the front office staff when patients call, as they must determine if the patient has a bundled, package, service plan, or fee for service. Attention to detail is necessary as some patients will pay for supplies, others have prepaid. All of these specifics are documented in the office system software, but Dr. Robbins cautions one "must have office personnel who can and do utilize that information." The practice is careful during their initial visit when reviewing insurance benefits to be sure patients understand there is "no guarantee of insurance benefit" until a claim is filed. On the rare occasion when the claim is processed differently than expected (and Dr. Robbins has confirmed it was processed correctly), the patient is billed for whatever balance is the patient's responsibility. In efforts to under-promise or over-deliver, Dr. Robbins has moved to a more generic "Insurance Estimate Form" that allows patients to review possible coverage scenarios. Dr. Robbins will have the patients initial each scenario as it is reviewed and they are given a copy of the form. As insurance policies have changed, this office has been able to be flexible and change with them. Dr. Robbins is able to follow the guidelines and rules of their contracts and still provide excellent care and service to each patient. They are also able to offer higher level technology instruments when patients request it.

Audiology Experts has been unbundled since 2011 and reports both the practice and the patients have had an extremely positive reaction to itemizing. As of March 2016, the practice reported that almost one hundred percent of all patients chose the service agreement the first year. During the second year, they had a ninety-seven percent renewal rate. Dr. Robbins shared that her profits increased seventy-nine percent as she moved from 2011 to 2014 (Robbins, 2016).

Comprehensive Care

Itemizing can serve the audiology professional and the patients quite well. Itemizing shows the patient what you have done. If you choose to continue to offer a "bundle" of your services, consider detailing for the patient the breakdown of all of the costs. There are indeed some patients who prefer the peace of mind that an all-inclusive plan offers. But even an "all-inclusive plan" should highlight that the patient has purchased hearing aids and your expertise.

As you contemplate how itemizing might work for your clinic, here are some suggestions that will get everyone in your practice thinking about their value:

- Assess the services you are providing your patient at each visit and determine if it is truly a pre-paid service.
- Employ the use of a superbill with each patient visit. Select all services provided during the visit regardless of whether there is a charge and send the patient home with a detailed itemization of all services provided. If the service is part of a service plan, indicate so on the invoice to dispel the notion that what you did was free.
- If your clinic is not presently utilizing the AAA Task Force Guidelines for the Management of Adult Hearing Impairment when fitting amplification, contemplate how to do it so it can add value to your practice and justify charging your service charges. The clinical practices outlined in these guidelines will set you apart from the competition and demonstrate your worth.
- Continue to educate yourself at professional meetings like AudiologyNow!, the Academy of Doctors of Audiology national meeting, your state professional meeting, and through reading journal articles. Stay current with best practice procedures as well as coding and billing and your insurance contracts. One must stay well-informed on what is happening in the profession and remain open minded to new ideas.

References

American Academy of Audiology. (2006). Guidelines for the Audiologic Management of Adult Hearing Impairment. Retrieved on October 27, 2014 from www.audiology.org /resources/documentlibrary/Documents/haguidelines .pdf.

Blackwell, D.L., Lucas J.W., Clarke T.C. (2014). Summary health statistics for U.S. adults: National Health Interview Survey, 2012. National Center for Health Statistics. Vital Health Stat 10(260).

Foltner, K. (2009). What's my time worth? Part 3: Breakeven analysis. *Advance for Audiologists*, 11(3), 44.

Gitles, T. (1999). Re-inventing the profession: A new model of hearing care delivery (First of two parts). *Hearing Journal*, 52(9), 32–34.

Gitles, T. (1999). Re-inventing the profession: A new model of hearing care delivery (Second of two parts). *Hearing Journal*, 52(10), 53–55.

itemize. (n.d.). *Dictionary.com Unabridged*. Retrieved October 1, 2015, from Dictionary.com website: http://dictionary .reference.com/browse/itemize.

Nemes, J. (2004). To bundle or not to bundle? That is the question. *Hearing Journal*, 57(4), 19–24.

Oden, L. (2016). Personal email communication. February, 28, 2016.

President's Council of Advisors on Science and Technology (PCAST). Aging America & Hearing Loss: Imperative of Improved Hearing Technologies [letter report to President Obama]. October 26, 2015. Retrieved on October 26, 2015 from https://www.whitehouse.gov/sites/default /files/microsites/ostp/PCAST/pcast_hearing_tech_letter report_final.pdf.

Robbins, K. (2016). Personal email communication. March 1, 2016.

Sjoblad S., Warren B. (2011). Mythbusters: can one unbundle and stay in business? *Audiology Today* 23(5), 36–45.

Sweetow, R. (2007). Instead of a hearing aid evaluation, let's assess functional communication ability. *Hearing Journal*, 60(9), 26–31.

Sweetow, R. (2009a). Hearing aid delivery models: Part 1 of 2. *Audiology Today*, 21(5), 49–57.

Sweetow, R. (2009b). Hearing aid delivery models: Part 2 of 2. *Audiology Today*, 21(6), 33–37.

Van Vliet, D. (2003). In praise of unbundling. *Hearing Journal*, 56(4), 36.

unbundle. (n.d.). *Dictionary.com Unabridged*. Retrieved October 1, 2015, from Dictionary.com website: http://dictionary .reference.com/browse/unbundle.

CHAPTER 6

Practicing in an Otolaryngology Office: Understanding Your Role in the Revenue Cycle

Kimberley J. Pollock

If you've chosen to work in an otolaryngology practice, it's not enough that you provide excellent clinical care and treatment to the patients referred to you by the physicians. By joining a practice, you've become an intricate part of a larger and more complex business that likely serves a wider range of patients than if you had chosen to open your own practice.

A core part of keeping this business, or any health care practice, *in business,* is how effectively it manages revenue cycle and reimbursement. The information you collect, your knowledge of coding, payer rules, and billing processes, and your use of charge capture tools and software systems all impact the practice's ability to get a claim out the door and be paid in a timely manner. And as the clinical provider in charge of the practice's audiology and hearing aid services, it's your responsibility to ensure that all these services are captured, appropriately coded, and submitted for billing.

Not only does this include the portion of services that are reimbursed by insurance plans, it also includes collecting patient financial responsibilities at the time of service. Although you may not be the one performing the charge capture keystrokes or asking for patient payment, your role is to make sure that the people and processes are in place in order to get these things done—or, to work with the practice's manager to facilitate. To be an effective leader in this role requires you to have an overall understanding of how to capture charges, code and document for them appropriately, and follow the correct procedures to bill for and collect from patients.

This chapter will give you an overall understanding of the revenue cycle in an otolaryngology office. It provides the knowledge, best practices, and modern technology information necessary to effectively bill and collect for audiology services in a practice. Even if you're still considering, or have already opened a private practice of your own, many of the recommendations in this chapter will apply to you as well.

Understanding Revenue Cycle Basics

Simply put, *revenue cycle* is a process that includes all the steps required to get medical, surgical, or audiology services paid. Figure 6–1 provides an overview of these for audiology services in most practices. If even one of the steps is overlooked or delayed, it creates a chain reaction that can result in a rejected claim, an uncollected patient balance, or even a full write-off of what could have been collected, had that step been completed correctly.

The revenue cycle is a process that includes all steps required for a practice to be paid for delivering audiology services. Other steps necessary in

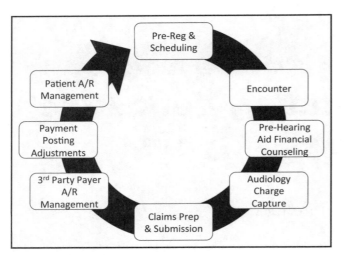

Figure 6–1. Steps in the practice revenue cycle.

an otolaryngology practice revenue cycle include pre-surgical counseling and surgery scheduling.

An audiologist's role in the revenue cycle is most vital at the Encounter and Charge Capture stages. You can help a practice avoid the Patient Accounts Receivable (A/R) Management step al-

together if you make sure copays and other patient financial responsibilities are collected before the patient leaves. That might even mean walking the patient to the check out desk so that the patient services representative can collect the patient responsible portion of the charges before the patient leaves the office. Many offices offer multiple payment options such as automated, recurring payments by credit/debit card, and patient financing programs for hearing aids, such as those offered by CareCredit or Wells Fargo.

Whether you are an employee or an independent contractor, your participation in the steps of the revenue cycle process will be the same. Table 6–1 provides an overview of an audiologist's role in practice revenue cycle.

Revenue cycle has both "front end" and "back end" processes (Table 6–2). Contrary to what you may think, *the most common billing mistakes don't actually happen in the billing office*. Most of them happen on the "front end" of the process, by the staff that schedules appointments, registers patients, and checks out patients in the office. That might be someone in the practice's central appointment

Table 6–1. Overview of the Audiologist's Role in Practice Revenue Cycle

Effective audiology providers participate in the revenue cycle of a practice in the following ways:

- Participate in the development of charge capture tools, templates, and forms specific to audiology services.

- Be diligent about making sure patients are registered and scheduled appropriately before performing diagnostic testing, as well as obtaining necessary precertification or referrals mandated by the insurance company. Without these plan "permissions," the payer may not reimburse the practice for the unauthorized services you may have provided.

- Know how to use electronic systems to capture and report charges, and document your services.

- Maintain current knowledge about CPT, ICD-10-CM, and HCPCS II coding for audiology services.

- Provide correct diagnosis codes to support tests and services performed, and perform adequate documentation to support them.

- Ensure that all billable charges are captured—including unscheduled ("add-on") services and tests, such as an audiogram and/or a tympanogram. Either reconcile the charges to the appointment schedule daily yourself or hold staff accountable for accuracy.

- Stay up to date on payer medical policies, including Medicare Local Coverage Determinations (LCDs), specific to audiology and/or vestibular testing. Understand payer payment guidelines for essential services such as vestibular testing, making sure that patients receive appropriate information about their financial responsibility.

- Review with the practice manager key metrics and the accounts receivable report each month.

Table 6–2. Common Front End and Back End Billing Processes

Front-End Processes	Back-End Processes
• Schedule appointment and preregister patient • Verify insurance, and validate medical benefits as well as audiologic diagnostic testing and hearing aid benefits and manage referrals and physician orders • Check-in/verify demographic data • Conduct patient encounter—code and document • Coordinate tests/procedure • Check-out and collect at point of service	• Submit claim/send patient statement • Correct front-end edits and resubmit • Process and analyze payments • Manage denials/resubmit • Follow-up on overdue receivables (payer and patient)

scheduling area or perhaps it is a dedicated audiology services scheduler. Modern practices understand that "front end" processes must be fine-tuned and nearly pitch perfect if the goal is timely and effective reimbursement.

A common practice is that the front desk staff be held accountable for accurate registration, insurance eligibility, benefits, and referral verification, and point of service collections or payment plan setup. Or, the audiology division might be large enough to have dedicated staff. The point is that this is a big shift in mindset from the "we'll bill you after insurance pays" culture that practices have held to for decades.

An Effective Revenue Cycle Is Front-End Focused

In our firm's work with otolaryngology practices, we find that *front-end billing processes are where most billing mistakes are made.* The root causes of claim denials and uncollected patient financial responsibilities can usually be traced back to the point that the appointment was scheduled, or the patient was seen in the office, and common denials include:

- Patient's plan does not include the audiologic diagnostic testing service or hearing aids as a benefit.
- Patient has an unmet deductible/coinsurance.
- Patient's copay was not collected.

- Patient did not have a referral for the diagnostic testing on the date of service.
- Patient was not eligible for insurance coverage on the date of service.
- Prior authorization for the diagnostic testing was not obtained.

Why are so many mistakes made on the front end? Often, it's because of these cultural norms:

- Front desk staff does not understand that they are part of the billing and collection process.
- Rejected claims and unpaid patient bills are perceived as the billing office's fault, so front desk staff is not held accountable.
- Front desk staff is not given the tools or the training necessary to do their job well.
- The front desk is perceived as an entry-level job so it may be filled with inexperienced, untrained individuals who are typically the lowest paid in the practice.
- The hearing aid evaluation scheduling process surprisingly does not include a notification to the patient that a deposit will be requested if not contractually prohibited.

Successful practices have changed the old front desk and scheduling culture to one that is proactive. They pre-register new patients and verify eligibility and benefits (e.g., diagnostic testing, surgical) prior to their arrival. They let patients know what will be collected, and that this may be more than their copay. Especially in an otolaryngology practice, where diagnostic scopes and cerumen removal are considered by many plans to be a "surgical procedure," staff let patients know that they will be asked to pay for their financial portion at the time of service. While many plans do not have mandatory copays for audiological diagnostic testing, some do. Verification of benefits prior to the appointment is important so that copays can be collected at the time of service and the practice does not have to wait for the patient payment after insurance has paid.

Service-focused practices also offer payment plans and patient financing to those who need a little extra time paying their bill. If the practice you work for does not, you'll be wise to suggest this—it's especially helpful for audiology and hearing aid patients, who have higher out-of-pocket responsibilities.

Audiologists can make the greatest impact on the revenue cycle by proactively participating in the front end of the billing process. As a clinical provider, you know which services were performed for the patient and why. The practice needs you to choose the right CPT®, HCPCS II, and ICD-10-CM codes for the patient. You can also insist that staff be trained about payment at the time of service rules. For instance, some plans have copays for diagnostic testing, *in addition to* the patient's office visit copay. Frequently, these go uncollected at the time of the visit, resulting in a practice sending statements for $15 or $20. This is expensive for the practice, and can be avoided if the team knows the rules and collects from the patient before he or she leaves the office.

The seven vital components of a well-managed front end process are described below. Understanding them is the audiologist's first step to making sure they are completed.

1. Set expectations on the first phone call. Appointment schedulers have an important role to play beyond just scheduling the appointment. They can set expectations about the correct documents to bring to the appointment and the types of services you provide. They can also let patients know they will be asked for payment for services rendered—not just their visit copay—and remind Medicare and managed care patients about referral requirements or that a second appointment might be nec-

essary if their referral does not include permission for audiology diagnostic testing.

2. Pre-register new patients. Pre-registration means obtaining complete patient demographic and insurance information and entering it into the computer system prior to the first visit. We have advocated this for decades and today it's more important than ever. That's because complete information is essential for ensuring the practice verifies insurance eligibility and benefits, knowing what the practice can collect from the patient in the office, and understanding referral or precertification requirements before a visit, test, hearing aid benefits, or surgery.

Patient portals, which allow patients to go online and register themselves, are a best practice way to pre-register because the data is automatically entered into your practice management system (PMS). Other options include calling the patient and pre-registering by phone, or emailing the forms to new patients in advance. Some practices include registration forms on their website.

3. Verify insurance eligibility and benefits, for new *and* established patients. It amazes us just how many practices skip this critical billing step. Or, they verify for new patients but not for established patients, only to find that the established patient is no longer eligible for the plan on record—which results in a rejected claim.

Before the Internet, eligibility verification took a lot of staff time on the phone. Today, many PMSs and electronic health records (EHRs) can be scheduled to perform these checks automatically, 48 to 72 hours prior to the patient's appointment. The system produces a report that indicates which patients are eligible and which are not. If done several days in advance of the patient's appointment, staff can call ineligible patients and explain that they will be responsible for paying for the visit. Front desk staff can also use the report to collect from ineligible patients or give them the option of rescheduling. If the practice's PMS doesn't have this "batch eligibility" feature, when the patient checks in, nearly all PMSs have a way to verify eligibility in real-time.

4. Obtain required managed care referrals for all new patients. Depending on the size of the practice, referral management can be performed at the time of appointment scheduling, or can be a separate

process. If a patient arrives for a hearing test or other audiology service without a referral, obtain it before they are seen or reschedule the patient. If you don't, the practice most likely will not be paid—or at the very least, payment will be delayed.

5. Precertify non-routine audiology tests. Insurance plans might require precertification for testing and services such as electronystagmography (ENG) or videonystagmography (VNG), auditory brain stem response (ABR), oto-acoustic emissions (OAE), electrocochleography (ECoG), or vestibular evoked myogenic potentials (VEMPs). Since many patients will require further diagnostic testing after being seen in the office, obtain precertification prior to the patient's arrival.

6. Verify patient identity, demographics, and insurance at check-in. The front desk staff plays a vital role here by validating the patient's identity and any previously obtained insurance information. Yet, this step is frequently overlooked due to the fact that the check-in staff is often overwhelmed with phone calls, chart prep (which must be done even with an electronic medical record), appointment scheduling, and check-in tasks. It's best to set up the front desk reception team for success by minimizing multitasking and allowing them to focus on verification tasks.

7. Collect from patients at the time of service. This means collecting more than just the visit copay. As patient responsibilities continue to rise, there is more to collect from patients than before as many Accountable Care Act (ACA) insurance exchange options have deductibles of $5,000 or more. As an example, deductibles for plans in Illinois range from $2,000 to $6,000.

   Setting expectations about what patients are expected to pay should be done on the first phone call. Research shows that patients appreciate knowing what they owe, as well as being provided options for settling their bill. According to a 2009 survey by McKinsey & Company, seventy-four percent of patients said they were willing and able to pay out-of-pocket expenses less than or equal to $1,000 and sixty-two percent were willing to pay medical bills greater than or equal to $1,000. Provide options and clear information, and collections will improve—especially if the practice implements up-front collection procedures. We believe that it's in the audiologist's best interest to ensure that

these procedures are followed for audiology services and, most especially, for hearing aid sales. Understand too that effectively collecting at the point of service does not work if all a practice does is tell the staff to "ask for money." Success requires a coordinated *plan* that includes:

- Clear financial policies for staff to follow.
- Technology tools that help them quickly identify the amounts they can collect.
- Scripts and talking points that help staff ask for money and handle patient objections.
- Training that ensures staff knows how to ask and collect effectively.
- A commitment from the physicians, audiologists, and the manager to review collections data and progress on a regular basis. Few things boost collections more than when staff is aware the physicians are paying attention.

What Does the Billing Team Do?

In the revenue cycle, the back-end processes are performed by what's commonly called "the billing department" or "reimbursement team." Unlike the front-end processes previously discussed, the back-end processes and tasks occur without direct contact with the patient. This makes the success of the team more challenging because, in our experience, the best chance for patient collections' success is when there is face-to-face contact with the patient.

In a best practice environment, the billing team does the following:

1. Reviews and verifies codes. In the most successful practices, physicians and other providers including audiologists—not coders, not EHRs—select codes. We have always been proponents of having the providers select codes because they are the ones delivering the service, and therefore know better than anyone what was performed. The billing team, however, must function as a knowledgeable "second pair of eyes" to ensure the codes selected comply with CPT® and ICD-10-CM rules as well as payer guidelines. The billing team's role is to verify accuracy and speak with physicians and other providers directly if changes are needed.

2. Submits claims electronically every day; this is, as they say, "billing 101." Successful practices submit accurate, "clean" electronic claims on a daily basis to as many payers as possible because they are processed faster than paper claims.

3. Reviews, fixes, and resubmits claims on the edit report—every day. We frequently find that this simple task goes undone in many offices. Here's what should happen: After the billing team transmits the day's claims electronically, the claims are reviewed or "scrubbed" by your electronic clearinghouse to ensure the demographic, insurance, and code information is appropriate before the claim is sent to the insurance company. This ensures that a "clean" claim is passed on to the payer. After the clearinghouse scrubs the practice's electronic claim batch, any missing demographic or insurance data that is missing is immediately sent back to the practice to correct. These are easy fixes—name, gender, date of birth—and can be completed quickly, which is why the review, fix, and resubmission of these claims must be done *daily*.

4. Speeds up payment posting with electronic payment remittance (ERA). ERA is a way to receive electronic payments directly into your practice management system. It decreases or eliminates the mundane staff task of posting payments all day at a computer.

5. Verifies electronic funds transfer (EFT) payments from payers. This is a staff efficiency tool that gets your money deposited into the bank account faster. Instead of receiving a paper check in the mail, payments from payers can be securely transferred to your practice's bank account using EFT, a one-way valve as funds can only be deposited and not removed. Using EFT reduces the number of checks your staff will have to deposit and fewer checks reduce the risk of employee theft. Most major payers offer the service, and there is no cost to enroll. In fact, it is required at the time of enrolling in Medicare.

6. Print and mail patient statements every day. Daily statement mailing is better for cash flow than waiting until month's end. Staff can generate patient statements immediately after a payment from the insurance company is posted. As point of service collections processes are implemented, the number of patient statements will be reduced. Alternatively, practices will engage the clearinghouse or some other third party to send patient statements. The point is that "best practice" is to get those patient statements out every day and not once a month.

7. Follows up on current balances quickly. Focus on unpaid claims in the "30-day" column of the accounts receivable report first. If staff stays ahead of the curve and gets the current claims paid quickly, in a short period of time, the number of "very old"(such as greater than 90 days) outstanding balances will be minimized.

8. Follow up on overdue claims and past due patient balances. In addition to focusing on the use of claim estimators and improving front-end collection processes, make sure there is an organized process for monitoring and following up on unpaid balances. To improve follow-up efficiency, staff should leverage modern payment technologies.

    For example, some clearinghouses offer claim status tools that enable staff to access online details about whether a claim was received by the payer and why the claim has not been paid. Not only does the use of such tools speed the follow-up process, it can eliminate the need for payer phone tag, handwritten notes, and the potential for staff to record verbally provided claim status details inaccurately. Staff login, use search and sort parameters to look up a patient's claim status, and obtain the details that are needed to understand status and take action.

    To follow up on past due patient balances, the billing team is empowered to establish payment plans, approve patients for charity care, and handle uninsured and underinsured patients who ask about cash discounts. Physicians as well as audiologists develop these policies, which the billing team implements and can manage with minimal oversight.

9. Verifies that payer payments are correct, according to contract. To make this efficient, billing staff enter all contracted payment schedules into the practice management system, and verify that payments match contracted amounts. Some systems do this automatically and alert staff to payments that don't match. Other systems require staff to review the payment amount against the payment loaded into the system.

10. Reviews and analyzes explanation of benefits (EOBs) forms received from payers. Appropriate analysis of each EOB is critical to ensure the practice was paid according to contract terms, and to drive the next steps in the revenue cycle, such as billing a secondary payer or sending a statement to the patient for payment of the balance. Another important aspect of EOB analysis is to determine any primary third-party claim follow-up, such as appealing services denied for inappropriate bundling, medical necessity, low pay appeals, incorrect coding, and inappropriate reporting of services during the global period.

EOBs are also a great diagnostic tool for evaluating whether billing processes are working. Ask for a sampling of EOBs for audiology services and have the billing team walk you through them to understand the data.

If you are an independently practicing audiologist, use the preceding information to develop a job description for the staff you hire. Screen them by asking about their experience in some of these areas, and be sure the candidate you choose can demonstrate experience and good references from previous otolaryngology and/or audiology employers. As an independent practitioner, the last thing you need to worry about is training someone who has a steep learning curve in billing. The ideal candidate would have prior otolaryngology/audiology billing experience, but this is not an easy skill set to find. At a minimum, the person you hire should understand billing processes and necessary tasks in the revenue cycle to ensure payments; specialty experience can be taught. Factor the cost of sending the new employee to otolaryngology and/or audiology-specific coding courses or webinars.

Revenue Cycle Metrics and Reports You Need to See. Revenue cycle metrics and diagnostic reports can help you understand the effectiveness of front end and other billing processes. Ask to meet monthly or quarterly with the practice manager or billing manager to review metrics, charges, collections, receivables, credit balances, and adjustments for the audiology department. Such data help you to understand the financial side of the practice, so that you can watch for reimbursement trends and resolve payment problems. Here is a list of metrics and reports to review as an audiologist in an otolaryngology practice or your own practice.

1. Revenue cycle metrics. Table 6–3 shows three key metrics to review regularly: Days in Receivable, Percent of A/R > 90 Days, and Net Collection Rate. Benchmark the practice data against the best practice metrics shown in the table.

    Days in receivable and percentage of A/R > 90 days are excellent metrics for measuring staff effectiveness and revenue cycle process efficiency. If these metrics are higher than best practice benchmarks, it means claims are taking longer to be paid, being denied—which requires correction and resubmission—or simply not being followed up on at all. High "days" and percentages > 90 days indicate a need for a deeper dive into what is going on, and fixing the issue at the source. When these metrics are "off," it's likely that front-end staff is not collecting accurate or complete data, patients are not being asked to pay at the point of service, and/or the code selection or denials management processes needs improvement. Most hearing aids involve a cash transaction, in which case you are paid the full fee; therefore, the Net Collection Rate will be 100% for those services and the Days in Receivable will be zero.

2. CPT® frequency. This is a standard report generated from the practice management system (Figure 6–2). Review it to understand hearing aid sales volume and the volume and types of audiology services you've delivered. Analyze trends by comparing the code data against the same month for the previous year, and year over year as well.

    The CPT® frequency report is standard in most practice management systems and allows audiologists to review service and product volumes to monitor increases and identify areas needing improvement.

3. Accounts receivable. This report shows total charges that have been billed and their aging status. As indicated in Table 6–3, receivables should stay as current as possible, with five percent or less over 90 days' old for audiology services. Physician services may take longer to be paid. Remember, hearing aid sales are usually a cash transaction, or benefits have been verified by a

Table 6–3. Key Revenue Cycle Metrics

	Key Revenue Cycle Metrics		
	Days in Receivable	**Percent of A/R > 90 Days**	**Net Collection Rate**
Description	The number of days, on average, it takes to get an account paid. To calculate: Total A/R Average Daily Charges* *Annual Charges/365	The percent of A/R that is at risk of becoming uncollectible. To calculate: Look at the 90 Day Column on A/R Report	The percent of collectible dollars that have actually been collected. Measures billing process effectiveness. To calculate: Total Receipts – Refunds Charges – Contractual Adjustments
Best Practice	20 to 30 days	15% or less	98% or higher

third-party payer prior to delivery, so there should be little to no outstanding charges for hearing aids.

4. Credit balances. Analyze the credit balance report monthly. Credit balances are those that your practice owes patients or insurance companies and you are required to refund them to the appropriate party. Credit balances are also a compliance issue. If an insurance plan or patient has overpaid the practice, *the practice must refund the overpayment*—regardless of whether plans or patients ask. Some payers, including Medicare, have specific deadlines for returning overpayments. The payers' guidelines should be investigated by the practice manager and followed. Such credit balances can often occur with hearing aids, when the patient pays up front and the insurance pays a portion after a claim was submitted.

Stay on top of these refunds by having the billing team generate a credit balance report monthly to review, validate, and submit a request for a refund to the practice manager or financial manager. Process refunds monthly; getting behind can become expensive. A 7-physician surgical practice had not generated the credit balance report for several years. When we did, it revealed more than $120,000 in credits that needed to be researched, validated, and potentially refunded.

Know the Reimbursement Rules. Billing is a detailed business, with reams of rules—from payer reimbursement guidelines and payment schedules to Medicare transmittals and code changes. Most of this information is readily available, but requires time and effort to locate, collect, organize, maintain, and update. If you or someone on the staff isn't paying attention to audiology service payer rules, the practice will experience a rise in claim rejections and receivables.

For example, audiovestibular testing is covered under Medicare's "other diagnostic tests" guidelines and not "Incident-to Billing" guidelines. Also there is no provision in the law for Medicare to pay audiologists for therapeutic services, only diagnostic testing services. Some Medicare Administrative Contractors (MACs) have a policy related to medical necessity for audiologic and/or vestibular testing while others do not. This is an example of why audiologists must have an understanding of both national and local carrier rules for the services they deliver. There are two guidelines that include this information: National Carrier Determination (NCD) and Local Carrier Determination (LCD).

If you simply followed national Medicare's NCD rule, yet your local carrier has a more restrictive policy for vestibular testing, the provider could be the cause of a lot of missed revenue for

ENT Associates
Audiology Service Codes
Jan 1 – Dec 31 2015
Provider: Anna Audiologist, AUD

CPT	Brief CPT Description	Frequency
92540	Basic Vestibular Eval	74
92542	Positional Nystagmus Test	0
92543	Caloric Vestibular Test	74
92545	Oscillating Pursuit Test	0
92547	Use of Vertical Electrodes	74
92550	Tympanometry and Reflex	86
92551	Screening Test, Pure Tone, Air Only	2
92552	Air Audiometry	33
92553	Air Bone Audio	1
92555	Speech Audiometry Threshold	2
92556	Speech Audiometry Threshold with Speech Recognition	3
92557	Comprehensive Audiogram	661
92565	Stenger Test Pure Tone	2
92567	Tympanometry	600
92568	Acoustic Reflex Testing	3
92570	Acoustic Immitance with Tympanometry	23
92579	Visual Reinforcement Audiometry VRA	113
92582	Conditioning Play Audiometry	4
92585	Auditory Brainstem Response, Comprehensive	80
92587	Otoacoustic Emissions, Limited	31
92588	Otoacoustic Emissions, Comprehensive	212
92591	Hearing Aid Examination and Selection, Binaural	1
92593	HA Check, Binaural	8
92620	Central Auditory Function, 60 min	2
92625	Tinnitus Assessment	50

Figure 6–2. Sample CPT® frequency report. *Note*: CPT® 92543 was deleted in 2016.

the practice. Further, the LCD for certain audiologic and/or vestibular testing services covers only certain ICD-10-CM diagnosis codes—and commonly used codes may not be covered. Audiologists need to know this in order to code correctly and submit an accurate claim—as well as what to do if the test doesn't identify the problem, or the local carrier does not cover the code for dizziness (R42).

Even five years ago, obtaining payer rules and guidelines required that staff make a lot of phone calls, and wait on hold for endless periods of time. This has changed significantly. Today, virtually every payer provides most if not all of their coding and claim submission guidelines, as well as provider manuals and reimbursement policies, online, but unfortunately this may not be true for hearing aid verification and benefits.

Collect Payer Guidelines. Start with Medicare, which publishes everything you need to know about submitting claims, billing, coding guidelines, how to bill for audiology services (https://www.cms.gov/Medicare/Medicare-Fee-For-Service-Payment/PhysicianFeeSched/audiology.html), National Correct Coding Initiative Edits (NCCI), and much more at www.cms.gov. Each year in the fall, Medicare publishes the full payment schedule that will be implemented the following calendar year. That's available on this site as well—as are many e-newsletters and webinars on key topics and upcoming changes. Sign up for all e-newsletters and attend webinars, and share what you learn with the practice manager, your colleague audiologists, and the practice team. Follow the information offered by your professional organizations, especially around the end of the year.

Next, gather audiology services policies from your MAC. The MAC is the organization that pays or denies Medicare claims, so your practice must know the details of how to appeal denials and request redeterminations when a claim has been rejected that you think should not have been. MACs generally follow Medicare rules, but not always. You must know the deviations for the services you deliver. While some private payers might cover hearing aids, Medicare does not so this scenario will always be a "cash" service.

After Medicare, conduct similar fact-finding missions at the websites of commercial payers and Medicaid. Nearly all of them provide medical policies, which is where you'll find essential information such as which ICD-10-CM codes are covered diagnoses for certain procedures, and hearing aids—the reimbursement rules for which vary widely by payer. With regard to managed care contracts, in an otolaryngology practice, reimbursement for diagnostic services performed by the audiologist can vary widely, and are all based on the managed care contract the practice has signed.

Each commercial payer and state Medicaid plan might also have a different policy for hearing aid coverage. There is no consistency across payers for hearing aid coverage in the United States; this is why verification of insurance benefits for non-Medicare patients is so important. For those payers who do provide coverage for hearing aids, it is important to ask more specific questions such as:

- What is the maximum dollar amount of coverage? Can you balance bill the patient for the difference between the covered amount and your fee?
- What specific type of hearing aid is covered?
- Can you bill the patient for the difference if they choose an "upgraded" hearing aid that is not covered by the payer?

Audiologists must pay particular attention to any benefits or coverage for hearing aids, and may need to involve a healthcare attorney in these discussions. Because the hearing aid that an insurance company covers may not be the right one for the patient, or the company may not reimburse enough to cover the actual cost of the hearing aid, knowing the details is important, and legal counsel is advised, especially when reviewing contracts.

Understand Contract Details and Audiology-Specific Billing Rules. When you join a practice, put your investigator's hat on and ask the following questions for all contracts the practice has signed. Knowing these rules is absolutely essential to your ability to assess the potential financial success of your audiology practice as well as to bill and collect from patients correctly. The most important thing to remember is that every rule, every reimbursement, and every form can vary widely from payer to payer. Knowing the rules can mean the difference between getting the practice paid in full or not being paid at all.

- Which audiology services are covered under the contract?
- If services are not covered, what can be collected from the patient as "non-covered?"
- If hearing aids are covered, which model or models are covered? Or, what is the amount covered? Is it a percentage?
- If insurance pays below the cost of the hearing aid, is the practice allowed to bill the patient the difference? What are the balance billing requirements?
- Are there specific disclosures that patients must sign? Are waivers allowed?

If you provide services to hospital patients, pay attention to *place of service* (POS) when you perform testing on a hospital patient who has been brought to the office. If the patient has Medicare, the carrier won't pay the claim if the billing staff selects the POS they typically use for office services, which is POS 11. A savvy audiologist will proactively let the billing staff know that the POS is *inpatient* so the staff can work with the hospital and/or investigate with the MAC the appropriate billing technique. Typically, diagnostic testing performed on an inpatient is included in Medicare's payment to the hospital through the diagnosis-related group (DRG) reimbursement. Make sure you understand other payer requirements for inpatient testing as well.

Offering newborn screening in the hospital is obviously a great way to detect early hearing loss and is also a good way to build visibility with pediatricians as well as increasing practice revenue. But before you see your first patient, get the payer-specific details about how to bill and get paid for these services. Follow these tips:

- *Research with your payers whether they will reimburse if the service is billed directly or if the service is included in the hospital payment.*

If the latter, you'll need to contract with a hospital for your services (e.g., per patient rate, hourly rate).

- *Obtain the patient's demographic information before performing the test.* Ask the practice billing staff to do this, if possible, as they'll need it for billing. Because the newborn patient will not be in the computer system, it is likely the parents won't be either.

  If the billing staff doesn't obtain the demographics, you could pull the face sheet from the hospital EHR after performing the service, or take a photo of it and securely send it to your billing staff. However, both of these options have HIPAA implications. Talk with your practice manager or compliance officer about a HIPAA compliant way to transfer this information. Mobile applications such as maxRVU provide HIPAA compliant solutions for collecting this information, along with charge data, and transmitting it securely back to the office billing staff (Figure 6–3).

WAYS TO IMPROVE POINT OF SERVICE COLLECTIONS. Effectively implementing billing processes and point of service collections requires access to information, and this requires the use of free or low cost tools.

One such tool is the online *cost estimator*. It used to be nearly impossible to predict what could be collected from patients until an EOB came with the plan's payment. But today, cost estimators provide real-time data about what a patient owes (see Figure 6–3). Staff enters the CPT® codes for office visits, audiological diagnostic testing, or hearing aids into the cost estimator, and the cost estimator calculates exactly what staff can collect for these office services.

The information supplied by the estimator depends on the patient's plan type, as well as the type of services entered. But generally speaking, a cost estimator allows a practice to calculate a patient's estimated patient responsibility based on his or her eligibility and benefits. Cost estimators are available through a clearinghouse such as Availity (www.availity.com), which offers them for free, as do many payers.

With deductibles and other patient financial responsibilities rising, patient financing is an appreciated option for many patients. CareCredit

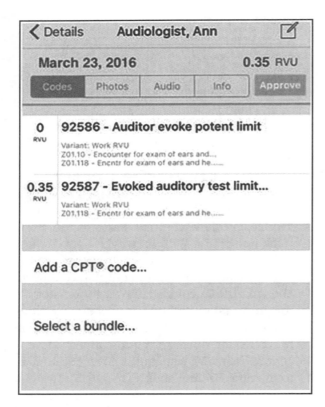

Figure 6–3. HIPAA-compliant mobile charge capture tools such as maxRVU by gingerCube. Inc. make collecting and transmitting demographic information from the hospital easy and secure. maxRVU improves the efficiency of the billing process by enabling secure messaging and document sharing between the provider and the billing staff.

(www.carecredit.com) is one option and there are others. This company offers a healthcare credit card that allows patients to finance large deductibles, coinsurance, and hearing aids, once approved. CareCredit offers 6- and 12-month no interest programs, as well as longer-term financing options. For a small service fee, a practice receives its money in two business days. CareCredit assumes the credit risk and handles the collections with the patient directly.

KEEP YOURSELF UPDATED AND EDUCATED. As Benjamin Franklin wisely said, *"An investment in knowledge always pays the best interest."* When it comes to billing and collections, this could not be truer.

Here's what we recommend for audiologists who want to stay current on coding and reimbursement topics:

1. Ask for an annual practice management/coding training budget for yourself. An appropriate request for an audiologist is around $1,500 per year.
2. Request a new CPT® book, or access to current CPT® resources, every year. Include ICD-10-CM and HCPCS II code books to your library as well.
3. Attend audiology or other specialty specific coding and reimbursement workshops. Not only will you get coding updates, you'll also meet and learn from other participants experiencing similar issues in their practices. Specialty societies, such as the American Academy of Audiology (AAA), the American Speech-Language-Hearing Association (ASHA), or the Academy of Doctors of Audiology (ADA), are the best options.
4. Sign up for webinars. Medicare, clearinghouse companies, and payers offer valuable education for free, online. Encourage others on the team to attend with you so you can discuss what you have learned. Again, your specialty societies are the first choices as education options.
5. Sign up for e-newsletters. There are many online resources available for free including your specialty societies. We suggest the following: CMS .gov, asha.org, audiology.org, and audiologist.org.
6. Be a leader for learning and sharing in otolaryngology/audiology practice staff meetings. Suggest to the practice manager that he or she divide learning opportunities among the staff and have participants summarize what they have learned for the group. This should be done in conjunction with the audiologist—coding, billing, and reimbursement for audiology services is a joint effort! This enables your team to participate in more webinars and workshops than if everyone had to attend all of them, and empowers staff who do attend to distill and teach-back the information to colleagues. When all teach, all learn.

Billing is a detail-laden and critical component of practice management. Audiologists must understand the basics and actively participate in coding and billing processes so that the practice is properly paid and is successful. The information presented in this chapter supports appropriate billing processes and healthy cash flow.

CHAPTER 7

Practice Management for Audiologists

Debra Abel

Introduction

In the preceding chapters, many tools for audiology practices have been provided by some of the profession's subject matter experts. Based on this infrastructure, this chapter will offer additional essential considerations for those contemplating the creation of an independent private practice or an autonomous practice affiliated with other audiologists, otolaryngologists, or other health care providers. The topics below are not a comprehensive list, but are to serve primarily as a checklist to assist with achieving your goals.

Essential Considerations for Establishing an Audiology Practice

Mission and Vision Statements

Both of these practice statements should be created for two reasons: For your staff to maintain focus and provide the pathway to a common purpose and also for those to whom you will provide services so they know what is important to you, how it will benefit them, and what is distinctive about your particular practice. Usually a few short sentences, the vision statement verbalizes the beliefs and dreams for the future, the uplifting tenants that will govern your practice. A mission statement is more concrete, shorter, and outcome-oriented

and describes the how's and why's of a practice. An online search will offer many examples of how to create both of these. Looking at other businesses' mission and vision statements may prove to be helpful for sentence structure and concepts.

Once created, these can be used for marketing, strategic planning, and may be a part of or separate from your practice's tag line, a short slogan that dramatically captures your practice's intent.

Professionals on Your Team

Attorney

Hiring an attorney familiar with federal and state health care laws is one of the first steps when forming a private practice. While this legal specialty may be more of a challenge to locate than others, there are several ways to do so. Contact your own primary care provider and/or your local hospital to see whose legal services they utilize as well as seeking suggestions from your local county bar and/or medical societies. At least one of these recommendations should lead to finding an attorney. You may want to interview several to ensure that they will be a good fit for your office and are knowledgeable about health care and those requirements specific to audiologists.

Whomever you choose needs to have a clear working knowledge of the federal and state regulations noted in Dr. Lewis' chapter (Anti-Kickback

Statutes, Safe Harbors, and Stark Laws), any business associate agreements you may need to create in order to be in compliance with HIPAA, as well as those specific state regulations that affect an audiology practice such as state Anti-Kickback Statutes, requirements of your state's insurance commission or department of insurance, and, of course, state licensure laws that pertain specifically to your state license and to your office. Local laws that apply to an audiology practice also need to be included. While the False Claims Act is a federal program, there may be similar state policies that also apply and are just as stringent. Also, attorneys can assist with corporation structure documents and provide guidance on which one may be the best direction for your practice. Finally, if you decide to contract with third-party payers, you will want to have those contracts reviewed by your legal counsel prior to signing on the dotted line.

Another first critical thing to do is obtain your own Tax Identification Number (TIN)/Employer Identification Number (EIN) at https://www.irs.gov/businesses/small-businesses-self-employed/apply-for-an-employer-identification-number-ein-online. You may need to register the name of your new practice in your state to ensure there are no duplicates. Other tax and city permits may be necessary. Your attorney can assist with obtaining any necessary state forms of registration, corporation, and state and federal tax structures, likely in tandem with your accountant.

Accountant

The services of an accountant are also an essential part of any practice and they can assist with recommendations regarding the corporate structure, tax benefits (state and federal), and also with profit and loss statements as well as other reports to ensure stability and growth. They can also make recommendations about your specific banking needs.

Budget projections and a business plan will also need to be developed and both of these professionals can offer input. There are many online resources, including the Small Business Association, which can assist with the creation of these documents, something necessary to complete before visiting with the next professional, your banker.

Accountants can also recommend a payroll company which can assist with payroll, payroll deductions including federal and state taxes, social security withholdings, and health care. These companies will generate reports for you as well as the W-2s you will need for any employees.

Banker

A personal banker is another professional you will need on your team, especially at the onset of building a practice. They can assist with opening the appropriate accounts for you that should include, at a minimum, a checking account and a line of credit for equipment purchase purposes or for times when revenue may be slower in arriving to your account. It is important to have a relationship with this professional as well so they may assess your practice needs and offer services specifically directed to your operations and growth.

Location

The old adage of "location, location, location" can't be understated when choosing the physical location of your practice. Of course it will depend on whether the space will be created due to a buildout or whether you decide to move into an existing space. You may need to secure the services of an architect/project manager and/or interior designer, depending on location and desired accouterments and, of course, the lease to be reviewed by legal counsel. Permits and licenses can be procured by the building professionals who should be familiar with local, state, and federal requirements. An office should have, at minimum, adequate parking, including several handicapped parking spots, an accessible path to and from the office, accessible restrooms, and other requirements of the American Disabilities Act. Costs will vary for whatever option is chosen, but each item should be included in a project estimate if doing a buildout or for those moving into an existing space, whatever is necessary to update it for your practice.

The name of your practice and signage are required to be an exact match as this may be monitored by federal payers due to the incidence of fraud and abuse. Having the practice name correspond exactly on all federal Internal Revenue Service and state tax documents as well as Medicare and Medicaid enrollment paperwork is vital.

The lease for your space should define which party is responsible for each of the utilities (gas, electric, sewage, Internet, trash removal, and water), snow removal and lawn care as well as hallway and restroom maintenance. For those items such as hallways and public restrooms, these may be included in the common area space shared by the others leasing offices in your building and may be expected to be paid monthly, semi-annually, or on an annual basis. This should also be itemized in your lease. Other inclusions that may apply to medical offices (e.g., call schedules and after-hours patient visits) may be included that don't apply to audiology, hence another reason for legal review to ensure that you can meet the requirements of your particular lease.

When procuring office space, it is necessary to be mindful of not only the physical appearance of an office, but also what is best for HIPAA compliance. If possible, a glass door separating the office from the waiting area is advised so that personal patient information is not overheard when patients make appointments or when financial information is discussed when they check out of the office when their services have been rendered. For those offices still utilizing hard copy paper charts, a locked file cabinet and a locked room are a necessity to protect Patient Health Information and not be in violation of HIPAA rules.

Licensure

At the time of press, every state in the United States requires an audiologist to be licensed either as an audiologist with hearing aid dispensing as part of that audiology license, as a dispensing audiologist, or for those states that require two separate licenses, a license for audiology and a separate license for hearing aid dispensing. Become familiar with the applicable laws and regulations in your state as these licensing bodies determine the scope of practice for service provision. If there is an incident and you are found to not be working within your scope of practice, there will likely

be some type of penalty that can run the gamut from a cease and desist, to a fine, to the loss of your license. This will be reported on your licensure record and depending on the severity, may also be reported to the national data bank.

Operating Management Systems (OMS)

A handful of operating management systems is available specifically for audiologists. It is encouraged that you interview each one to see the best fit for your office needs. Be mindful that the future will likely be a paperless office with all billing submissions and patient records electronic. Some of these OMS have modular capacities, so that you can begin with a basic package and upgrade as your needs change.

Equipment

The following equipment listed below is necessary for a diagnostic and dispensing audiology practice. Those with asterisks are essential in order to provide minimal services. As a practice becomes more established, additional capital can be included in your annual budget to prepare for additional purchases which may include adding additional services such as vestibular testing and treatment and cerumen management. Your equipment distributor can offer return on investment (ROI) information so that you know how many tests you need to complete and how often in order to pay off the equipment within an established time frame when deciding on future purchases. You can also inquire about leasing options with your distributor.

Office Equipment

- Computer and peripherals (software, modem, printer/scanner)*
- Office management system for scheduling appointments, filing claims, billing, invoicing*
- DVDs or thumb drives to back up information for offsite storage*
- Copier and fax machines*
- Phone system with voice mail*

- Sterilization equipment*
- Locked file cabinets if housing Personal Health Information*
- Fire extinguishers*
- First aid kit*
- Defibrillator* (may be required by law)

Office Furniture

- Desks for front office staff and tables for waiting area*
- Chairs for front office, booth, audiologist(s), and waiting area*
- Locked filing cabinets*

Office Supplies and Resources

- CPT®, ICD-10-CM, and HCPCS code books
- Business cards, appointment cards, and brochures with holders for each*
- Stapler and staples, tape, manila and business envelopes, stamps or postage machine, pens, pencils, pencil sharpeners, paper, paper clips, scissors, rubber bands, DVDs or thumb drives for back up storage, self-inking stamp with office name and address, and clipboards*
- Employee name tags (first names only)
- Frames for licenses and other required forms that need to be posted
- Paper shredder, wastebaskets, and garbage bags*
- Magazines for waiting area
- Display case for hearing aids/assistive listening devices
- Microbial soap and paper products (tissues, toilet paper, and paper towels)*
- "No smoking" sign as well as evacuation route posted in case of a fire (may be required by law)
- Notice of Privacy Practices in waiting area*

Audiometric Equipment

- Otoscopes and disposable speculum*
- Sound-treated booth (required by Medicare)*
- Audiometer with headphones or if insert phones, disposable ear tips*

- Tympanometer and ear tips*
- Otoacoustic emissions and ear tips
- Vestibular equipment if providing vestibular services and disposables/goggles
- Computer with NOAH* and other essential programs (Outlook, Word Document, Excel)*
- Manufacturer software, links, or cables*
- Visual reinforcers for Visual Reinforcement Audiometry
- Toys for Conditioned Play Audiometry
- Budget for annual calibration*
- Ear mold impression material, otoblocks, earlights, shipping boxes and labels for impressions, injection syringes or guns, ear mold reamers, and tubing blowers*
- Alcohol and other cleaners for sterilization*
- Cerumen removal management tools, suction, and magnification
- Hearing aid supplies (battery doors, hooks, domes, receivers, tubing, boxes and shipping labels, order and repair forms, superglue, tubing glue, tubing expander, Dremel drill, ultrasonic cleaner, Redwing, battery testers, battery removal tools)*
- Batteries for hearing aids*
- Flashlights in each room in case of a power outage
- Smoke and carbon monoxide detectors*
- Fire extinguisher*
- Gloves (avoid latex for those who may be allergic)

Staffing

A very new audiology practice often relies on just one person to do all necessary office services. With growth, new positions can be added in. If fortunate to begin with staff, the front office staff (FOS) is the window and door to your practice. This person should have the personality of an angel in order to be kind to patients and the converse, a devil, in order to collect payments from what can be difficult payers. This person sets the tone to your mission and vision and is the initial face to your practice. Necessary traits include good communication and people skills as there will be challenges presented.

Practices will also want to consider a BOS, or back office staff, for insurance verification and collections when the practice has reached a level of financial stability to hire a new staff member.

Training will need to be completed with each new office staff person as it relates to office policy, payment verifications, prior authorizations, and payment requirements. HIPAA reviews need to be done at the time of hire and annually. Some payers require fraud and abuse training for the entire staff and they will inform you when that training is to take place. Payments should be collected at the time of service unless there is a secondary co-pay that will need to be billed or if a contract disallows patient payments until they make their own restitution.

Finally and often overlooked is the need for cleaning personnel. While this could be the job of someone in the office, if affordable, hiring a local service will be appreciated by current staff.

Marketing

Marketing is one of the largest items that should appear in the annual budget and on a targeted marketing plan calendar. In the 2011 Hearing Review, Phonak noted that a medium practice spends 4.8 percent of gross revenue or about $15,000 annually and an average practice 7.3 percent or $61,514, respectively, with many variables determining what is spent and on what, including physician referrals, practice setting, and the goals of the practice.

In the last decade, changes from large Yellow Pages listings have transitioned to a website presence and ads in the local paper now also include social media. Direct mail, newspaper advertising, and outbound phone calls made by staff are still consistently and effectively utilized and many feel bring in a successful number of referrals when targeted at the correct audiences. Practice newsletters and community educational classes are also a contact point to update participants on new technologies and create or maintain a connection to your practice. One of the best and most inexpensive marketing tools is to send a thank you letter to the referring provider describing the patient's visit and recommendations. This should be done in the name of good patient care, especially for Medicare beneficiaries. Visits to nursing homes and senior centers are also options, depending on the demographics and needs of your community. Once you are established, cull your existing data base for those 4+ year patients who may be interested in new technology; clean and checks appointments are also a way to maintain the patient's loyalty and ensure that their needs are being met.

Demographic information can be purchased online and the local Chamber of Commerce may have access to the targeted demographic your practice would like to court. Expect to pay for this information and see what local colleagues and other health care professionals have found successful in their practice areas.

Brochures and business cards are a must, especially if you are providing information describing your services to your referral sources. Have a few in your waiting area so that satisfied patients can offer them to their friends and family.

Logo

In order to establish a practice identity, a logo should be created, so that when viewed, it will trigger a reminder of your practice to anyone who sees it. This is typically created as part of the marketing plan, often with a graphic designer who can also assist with the creation of your business cards, website, brochures, and other marketing materials.

Message on Hold

In the short time that patients wait on hold when they place a call to your office, having a message on hold is another marketing mechanism to educate your callers on the services provided in your practice. An Internet search can provide local companies who offer these services in your area.

Policy and Procedures Manual

A policy and procedures manual is essential for every practice to understand and manage expectations of what is required in the office workplace for the employee as well as for patients. At the very least, this should include the mission and vision statements, job descriptions for all positions, performance review forms, policies addressing paid time off, medical and family leave as required by law, continuing education, liability and licensure policies, hearing aid policies for purchase and collections, loss, damage, and repair. To create a comprehensive manual, the author strongly suggests reading Dr. Robert Glaser's Chapter 10 in *Strategic Practice Management: Business and Procedural Considerations*, Second Edition, a must for any practice, especially for those in their prenatal or infant stages.

Situations that will likely need to be addressed in your policy and procedures manual that are becoming much more common are for those devices obtained elsewhere, either from another practice, from an insurance payer, or from the Internet, and how these patients will be treated and how they will be billed for these types of services. A waiver attesting to their understanding of what is expected may also be helpful, but should be generated or reviewed by legal counsel.

Federal and State Regulations and Licensure Laws

Preceding chapters included the federal and state laws that must be followed when providing audiologic and vestibular services to patients. Ignorance is not an excuse, so you must be knowledgeable of the regulations, how these impact your practice, and follow them accordingly.

At press time, all audiologists in the continental United States, Alaska, and Hawaii are required to be licensed in the state in which they practice. Some states have an audiology license that also includes hearing aid dispensing by virtue of being an audiologist, some states have a separate and additional license with one for audiology and an additional license to fit hearing aids, and other states have a dispensing audiology license that allows for the provision of diagnostic service and hearing aid services provided by audiologists as well as an audiology only license that does not allow fitting hearing aids. You must be licensed in

order to provide services; your audiology license governs your scope of practice and professional behavior and it is incumbent upon each licensee to know the regulations and laws that govern the practice of audiology and hearing aid dispensing in the state in which they practice. If a question arises, contact your licensure board for an opinion and/or guidance.

Liability Insurance

There are two types of liability insurance required as a practice owner: Office liability and professional liability. Your office space must be insured for theft, fire, flood, calamity, and injury, something that can be obtained with a local insurance agent. If you are located in an area prone to national disasters, check to see if you can incorporate the time if the office is forced to close due to a disaster. If you don't have an insurance agent, your local Chamber of Commerce can assist with providing a list of agents in your area.

You must also have malpractice or liability insurance. The national audiology professional organizations as well as some of the state organizations offer reasonable plans. Most third-party payers require a minimum of $1,000,000/$3,000,000 coverage, typically the amount offered by these plans. For those who consult and teach, riders can also be added at an additional minimum cost.

Forms Necessary for an Audiology Practice

The following lengthy list is not exhaustive, but is to serve as a guide to those forms necessary in any practice. Pages 331 to 333 of *Strategic Practice Management: Business and Procedural Considerations*, Second Edition offers several as examples for ear mold impression taking and cerumen management waivers. The national audiology professional organizations also have forms for purchase or on their websites. For the list below, websites were provided, when possible, for you to create your own forms. It is suggested that your legal counsel review them to ensure they capture all possible scenarios and are in compliance with the laws that govern your practice.

- Notice of Privacy Practice (HIPAA) http://www.hhs.gov/hipaa/for-professionals/privacy/guidance/model-notices-privacy-practices/
- Advanced beneficiary notice (Medicare) https://www.cms.gov/MEDICARE/medicare-general-information/bni/abn.html
- Release of information
- Hearing aid/cochlear implant/osseo-integrated device loaner agreement (acknowledging when it was given, returned, and if loss or damage should occur once it leaves the audiology office)
- Hearing aid waiver (check your state licensure laws—as of December 2016, the waiver will no longer be enforced by the FDA for those age 18 and older): https://www.fda.gov/newsevents/newsroom/pressannouncements/ucm532005.htm
- Purchase agreement (many states have requirements of what is to be included in their hearing aid dispensing regulations, so check your state's website or contact your state licensure board for guidance)
- Hearing aid checklist (demonstrating to the patient how to insert and remove the device from their ear, how to insert and remove the battery and how it needs to be stored and the contraindications of batteries, other medical contraindications, how to care and treat the device, etc., with a copy retained in the chart and one given to the patient, signed and dated by both parties)
- Extended warranty agreement (may include clean and checks, in house repairs, manufacturer loss, damage, repair, and warranty policies)
- Superbill/encounter forms (available from the national professional organizations; a charge may be assessed) with the CPT®, ICD, and HCPCS codes utilized in your office

- Contracts with other offices, hospitals, and nursing homes to be reviewed by legal counsel prior to signing in the provision of offsite services

Establishing a Fee Structure

As already noted, it is critical to know your hourly rate in order to establish an office's fee schedule; otherwise, you may be undercharging for your services. Dr. Sjoblad outlined that well in her chapter and would refer you to the formulas she included when establishing your hourly rate and basing your fees on what that hourly rate plus desired profit is. For example, if it takes 45 minutes to perform a hearing evaluation and your hourly rate is $XXX.xx, then you could bill ¾ of your hourly rate plus your desired profit as the fee for this service and your usual and customary charge is $YYY.yy.

Third-Party Payers

The decision to contract with third-party payers must be weighed carefully. As noted in an earlier chapter, audiologists cannot opt out of Medicare and if the practice's decision is not to enroll in Medicare, then all diagnostic services to all patients are to be provided at no charge. Commercial payers' policies are different, but some adopt Medicare guidelines as well as require enrollment in Medicare as a proviso of being enrolled with them. Each patient must be billed the same amount for each item and service, regardless of the payer. What you will be reimbursed by the payers will be different based on the agreed upon fee schedule contained in your payer specific individual contracts. It is suggested that you incorporate your fee schedules for all payers in your office management system so that when payment is posted, the contracted rate and the payment rate should be identical, indicating that there are no errors in payment. It may be necessary to write off adjusted contractual fees and these should also be tracked. If the claim was poorly paid or not in accordance with the fee schedule, this should trigger an appeal, a process that should be detailed in your contract.

With many employers offering a hearing aid benefit, which sadly, is not one at all, it is critical to understand the contracts and these should be reviewed by legal counsel. Fee schedules need to be included to see if you do choose to sign on that you won't lose money and there are contracts where that will occur. Knowing your hourly rate is essential as well as knowing what the contract requires in terms of the device, the trial period, the number of rechecks, and the length of the warranty period that are required to be provided at no charge. Some require services for the life of the device and those will also need to be weighed for a practice's affordability.

For those patients who choose to upgrade to more premium technology, when verifying hearing aid benefits, the question should be asked of the payer if the patient can share in the cost of the upgrade, beyond their benefit. The payer should then be asked if the patient can sign a waiver and does that payer provide one or can the practice generate one. If the practice can generate one, it needs to include the patient's name, date of service, and what their financial responsibility is for this non-covered service. Their insurance reimburses for covered services and will likely be reflected as such on their Explanation of Benefits. All hearing aid benefits should be verified at the time of the hearing aid evaluation so that all parties are clear about their fiscal responsibilities, lessening heartburn and bad feelings that can impact the practice.

At press time, several major commercial payers were utilizing a third party to assume the cost of goods and, in turn, were paying the audiologist a fitting fee for professional services. These third-party payers reimburse a fixed amount for the fitting fee, rechecks, and other services, while some are discount programs only, meaning you provide the device and services and offer the patient the discount when required to do so. While it may be appealing for some practices to not have finances tied up in the cost of goods for hearing aids, if you are barely able to make a profit from

these plans, you will need to consider all aspects, positive and negative, when engaging in these contractual arrangements. Do not contract out of fear that you may lose patients, but based on data that includes the demographics of your practice area, what you can or can't afford to lose, and the future health of your practice.

Professional Dues

Part of maintaining awareness of what is happening in and to the profession and being heard are two important benefits of membership in national and state audiology organizations. There are many resources available to members on these organizations' websites. Membership fees need to be considered in the annual budget process.

Conclusion

While not an exhaustive list of considerations, these topics are essential suggestions for anyone contemplating the establishment of an autonomous independent private practice or one affiliated with other providers. As the future continues to evolve at what may seem an incredibly rapid rate with a perfect storm of disruptive technologies, government initiatives, and major retailers, these tools should provide the fundamental foundation, serving as the rudders in these uncharted waters.

References

Glaser, R. G. (2014). Policy and procedures manual. In R. Glaser and R. Traynor (Ed.), *Strategic Practice Management: Business and Procedural Considerations*, Second Edition (pp. 335–356). San Diego, CA: Plural Publishing.

Phonak. (2011). A survey of key metrics for benchmarking a hearing practice, Part 2. *Hearing Review*. 18, 24–30. Retrieved June 1, 2016 from http://www.hearingreview.com /2011/07/a-survey-of-key-metrics-for-benchmarking-a -hearing-practice-part-2/.

Index

Noise-induced hearing loss
   legal ramifications of, 40–45
   tort law for, 42–44
   Workers' Compensation programs for, 44–45
Non-covered service, 3, 12, 28–29, 47, 63–64, 67, 97, 106
NPI. *See* National Provider Identifier
Nystagmus, 3, 11, 7–8, 95

O

Occupational Safety and Health Act of 1970, 36
Occupational Safety and Health Administration, 36
Office equipment, 101–102
Office furniture, 102
Office management systems, 30, 101
Office supplies and resources, 102
OHCA. *See* Organized health care arrangement
OMS. *See* Office management systems; Operating management systems
Online cost estimator, 97–98
Operating management systems, 30, 111
Opting Out, Medicare 19, 24
Optokinetic nystagmus test, 7–8, 11
Order, 2, 19, 21–26, 64
Organized health care arrangement, 54
OSHA. *See* Occupational Safety and Health Administration
Osseointegrated services, HCPCS II codes for, 11–12
Ototechnicians, 30–31
Out of pocket expense, 64–65, 82, 90–91
Out-of-network, 64–65, 82
Overdue claims, 92

P

Past due patient balances, 92
Patient Protection and Affordable Care Act, 47, 91
Patient responsibility, 64, 79, 97
Patient statements, 92
Payable amount, 64
Payment schedule, 92, 94, 96
Payments, 30, 91–94, 102–103
PCAST. *See* President's Council of Advisors on Science and Technology
Penalties, 20, 26, 36, 45–48, 57
Percent of A/R > 90 Days metric, 93, **94**
Personal health information, 49–52, 57, 102
Personal supervision, 64–65
PHI. *See* Protected health information
Physician fee schedule, 7, 26, 30
physician orders (Medicare), 2, 19, 21–26, 64
Physician quality reporting system, 29–30

Place of service, 97
Point of service, 65, 89, 91–93, 97
Policy and procedures manual, 103–104
POS. *See* Place of service; Point of service
Positional nystagmus test, 7, 11, 95
PPACA. *See* Patient Protection and Affordable Care Act
PPO. *See* Preferred provider organization
PQRS. *See* Physician quality reporting system
Practice. *See* Audiology practice
Predetermination, 65
Preferred provider organization, 65
Pregnancy Discrimination Act of 1978, 38
Pre-registration, of new patients, 90
President's Council of Advisors on Science and Technology, 71
Primary insurance, 65
Prior authorization, 64–65, 89, 103
Privacy Rule. *See* HIPAA Privacy Rule
Private insurance, 61
Product noise labeling, 36
Products liability, 43
Professional dues, 106
Professional liability insurance, 7, 104
Professional malpractice, 45
Professional meetings, 84
Protected health information, 48–56
Provider, 26, 46–58, 62–69, 88, 91, 94, 96
Provider Enrollment Chain, Ownership System, 26–27
Provider Transaction Access Number (Medicare), 10
Punitive damages, 42
Purchase agreements, 105

Q

Quiet Enjoyment, 45

R

Radiologist, 25
Rapid eye movement sleep, 38
Reevaluation, 22
Referrals, 19, 46–48, 65, 88–91, 105
Rehabilitation Act of 1973, 40
Relative value unit for work, 6–7
REM sleep. *See* Rapid eye movement sleep
Renegotiation, of contract, 69
Revenue cycle
   audiologist's role in, 88
   back-end processes, 88, **89**
   basics of, 87–89
   billing team involved in, 91–93
   collecting payments from patients, 91

W

Wells Fargo, 88
"Whistle-blowing," 41–42, 46
Work relative value units
    for audiologic function tests, 8
    description of, 6–7
for evaluation and therapeutic services, 8–9
    for vestibular function tests, 7–8
Workers' Compensation programs, 44–45,
    61–62
Workshops, 98
"Worthless Service," 46–47
Write-offs, 65